tim anders‹

MW00807598

OS
PRESSING
RESET
original strength
reloaded

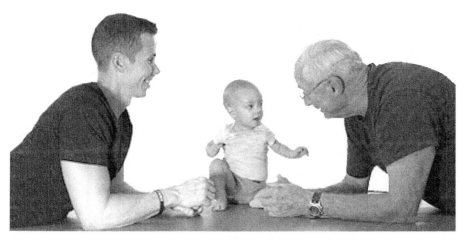

FONTLIFE PUBLICATIONS

Pressing RESET, Original Strength Reloaded
by Tim Anderson and Geoff Neupert

A FontLife Publication, LLC
Raleigh, NC 27603
http://fontlifepublications.com/

Edition ISBNs:
Softcover: ISBN-10: 1-62422-029-0
               ISBN-13: 978-1-62422-029-6
Kindle: ISBN-10: 1-62422-030-4
               ISBN-13: 978-1-62422-030-2

Second Edition 2015
Printed in the United States of America

Library of Congress Control Number: 2015952895

Original Cover Art by Danielle "Dani" Almeyda

Contents

Thanksgiving

<u>From Tim:</u>

Thank you, God. You made all of us to be strong and courageous. You have taught me how wonderfully designed I am, and how awesomely loving You are. I asked You to teach me how to become bulletproof and You did. Thank you. You are my *Original Strength. –Psalm 43:2*

To my wife, Addie, you are my queen. There are not enough words to express my heart and gratitude towards you. I am a blessed man. Thank you.

Geoff, Dani, John U, John B, and Trey: You are my family. I am eternally grateful for you all.

<u>From Geoff:</u>

Father, thank you! Without you, none of this would've been possible—I would've missed it all!

Tim, what can I say, you are Superman. Thanks for being my brother.

Courtney, my wife, thanks for putting up with my craziness. I love you.

Connie, Becker, Elliot, Aron, Minta, Bev, Lee, Eileen, Gary, Peter, and Marel: Thanks for the extreme privilege of working together all these years. You have been my "lab" and my "guinea pigs" and I thank you for trusting me to "test" out my theories. I'm glad this last one was the last one we'll ever need. I will miss you all dearly.

We would both like to thank the outstanding professionals who helped us see "outside the box:" Carla Hannaford and Sally Goddard Blythe and their outstanding work with children, reflexes, and movement. You gave us "eyes to see" what was missing in the health and fitness industry.

Disclaimer!

You must get your physician's approval before beginning this exercise program.

These recommendations are not medical guidelines but are for educational purposes only. You must consult your physician prior to starting this program or if you have any medical condition or injury that is contraindicated to performing physical activity. This program is designed for healthy individuals 18 years and older only.

See your physician before starting any exercise or nutrition program. If you are taking any medications, you must talk to your physician before starting any exercise program, including the *Original Strength* program. If you experience any lightheadedness, dizziness, or shortness of breath while exercising, stop the movement and consult a physician.

It is strongly recommended that you have a complete physical examination if you live a sedentary lifestyle, have high cholesterol, high blood pressure, diabetes, are overweight, or if you are over 30 years old. Please discuss all nutritional changes with your physician or a registered dietitian. If your physician recommends that you not use the *Original Strength* program, please follow your doctor's orders.

All forms of exercise pose some inherent risks. The authors, editors and publishers advise readers to take full responsibility for their own safety and know their limits. When using the exercises in this program, do not take risks beyond your level of experience, aptitude, training and fitness. The exercises and dietary programs in this program are not intended as a substitute for any exercise routine, treatment or dietary regimen prescribed by your physician.

Having said all of that, this is not an exercise book. The movements in this book are the movements you have already made, and they are the movements that you probably should be making every day. For example, we introduce breathing in this book. If your doctor advises against breathing, you should probably seek out another doctor, or at least ask for a second opinion!

There is a small exercise section in this book, but the book itself is intended to help you remember how you were designed to move. Again, this is not an exercise book. This is a movement restoration book. Enjoy!

Foreword

As someone who has incorporated *Original Strength* (OS) concepts into my practice as well as my own personal fitness, I have experienced its benefits first hand and witnessed it change the health and wellness of others. A few years ago, after a 16-mile trail run, I twisted my knee on dry creek bed. Afterward, I developed a recalcitrant knee pain that was confirmed on MRI as a chondral defect, a condition where permanent damage had been done to the cartilage in my knee. As I have always done with my patients, I took a very biomechanical approach to my problem performing many of the best evidence-based exercises, modifying activity, and nutritional supplementation. My strength improved, but joint mobility with deep knee flexion, dead lifts, and kettle bell swings along with pain during running were still problematic. Mark Shropshire, a trusted strength and conditioning coach, introduced me to Tim's early works, *Becoming Bulletproof* and *Original Strength,* and I began working on "The Big Five" over the course of the following year. Since that time, I have returned to recreational running, completing a marathon and have helped many others return to activities that they didn't believe were possible.

After having success with OS for my personal rehabilitation, my daughter incorporated OS into a strength and conditioning program as an athlete with the USA Luge Team. It is often said that luge races are won in the summer, not in the winter. The preparation that gives an athlete a fast, powerful start, strong neck muscles needed to maintain optimal aerodynamics, and core control to steer a sled down an icy track at 90 mph, is a learned practice during the off season.[1] It is the commitment to the fundamentals of rocking, rolling, crawling, head control, and breathing that the good athletes become great athletes and when the Olympic hopeful becomes the Olympian.

Often times, something that starts as a personal interest has a way of influencing our professional interest. In 2013, the American Physical Therapy Association's Vision Statement for the Physical Therapy Profession defined movement as "a key to optimal living and quality of life for all people that extends beyond health to every person's ability to participate in and contribute to society."[2] Working with recreational and professional athletes, corporate and medical executives, and people with differing abilities, those who perform well are those who are able to master the transition from one movement pattern to another, achieving a desired functional outcome. Tim Anderson has taken the fundamental principles of movement system development strategies we innately employ as infants and toddlers and has reintroduced them to us as adults in a systematic manner.

Motor learning or skills acquisition can be broken down into two main categories: sequence learning and sensorimotor adaptation.[3] Often times, when learning new motor patterns, we will break the complex sequence into its constituent components and gradually integrate each component into its sequence. Take for instance, crawling. It is a complex movement that incorporates stability, mobility, and strength of the upper and lower limbs, scapulothoracic complex, and the lumbopelvic complex. Yet those complex movements are predicated by our horizontal gaze, head position, and breathing. Our sensorimotor adaptations such as the absence or presence of visual inputs, applied resistance or unweighting, or contact pressures all influence our response to altered limb dynamics that are associated with crawling.

" I admire Tim's passion for helping others and trust you will enjoy reading his latest inspiration: Pressing RESET, original strength reloaded.

With the use of a hierarchical approach to standard movement patterns of diaphragmatic breathing, head control, rocking, rolling, and crawling, Tim has provided a simple methodology for the therapist or exercise specialist to progress or regress a movement sequence to optimize motor learning. As a physical therapist that treats primarily orthopedic conditions and sports-related injuries, I have come to appreciate the essential role that proper movement system development has on my clients' ability to optimize their quality *IN* life.

I am grateful that Tim has been inspired to develop and refine the concepts of *Original Strength*. I admire Tim's passion for helping others and trust you will enjoy reading his latest inspiration: *Pressing RESET, Original Strength Reloaded.*

– Ken Johnson
PT Manager, Outpatient Rehabilitation Therapy Services
Administrator, Johns Hopkins Hospital/George Washington University
Orthopaedic Physical Therapy Residency
Johns Hopkins Hospital
Baltimore, Maryland

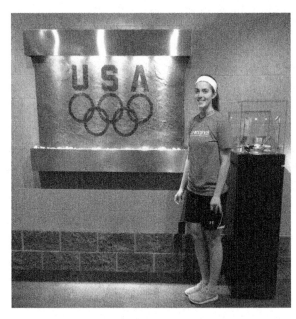

Camille Johnson, sporting OS shirt, at US Olympic Training Center in Lake Placid, NY 2/25/2015

The Beauty in the Simplicity

– Chip Morton,
Strength and Conditioning Coach, Cincinnati Bengals

In my 30 years as a professional in the strength & conditioning field, I have witnessed, studied, and even used many of the ideas, techniques, and trends that characterize the ebbs and flows of our industry. Strength, stamina, power, flexibility/mobility, and the desire to maintain an appropriate body fat percentage, have been, and likely always will be, important training goals for many people. Once during my first couple of years on the job as a strength coach in professional football, an older, more experienced coach told me that the most important aspect of a player's development to address in training was "movement". At the time, I dismissed it in favor of the more obvious responsibilities most often associated with my position, namely, strength and conditioning. Over the years, as I have matured and gained in wisdom and knowledge, my views have changed. I now understand and more fully appreciate the insight that older coach imparted to me years ago. We are in fact, "made to move."

Over the past few years, I have noticed a lot of attention and information has been devoted to helping people move *better*. We are told which mobility drills & stretches are best to perform and why, as well as how to perform them correctly; we're shown progressions, regressions, "flows", and the like. Within the variety of movement templates available on the Internet and in the literature, many are interesting to watch or read about. You can usually glean a few bits of usable information and even uncover common threads, or "truths", that weave their way through different programs. Some of the recommendations can be therapeutic, others may make you feel good, and even be fun to do. At some point, however, it seems to me, the more information we are presented with, the more complex things become, and the more difficult it is to discern what is best and how to put it all into practice on a consistent basis.

Moving well and what is required to attain that can be viewed from so many perspectives. There are many gifted individuals out there, demonstrating abilities forged from years of regular practice, perhaps with favorable leverages and the body dimensions necessary to master a particular skill set. As beautiful or enticing as they may appear, some movement prescriptions may not be a good fit for some people. This may stem from the amount of time and repetition required to achieve competency, or an inability to fit all the "moving parts" into an everyday schedule.

Finally, the prescription itself may simply not provide an appropriate entry point for certain individuals along their journey to reach their goals. The concept of "better movement" itself, is a quality unique to the individual to an extent, and lies along a continuum ranging from accessing the ranges of motion to improve day to day life, all the way to the ability to perform the movements required for elite athletic performance. Each one of us will define this quality differently, depending upon our individual needs and what we desire to accomplish.

The good news is God had already knit a movement "template" into each one of us. In fact, we progressed through parts or all of this progression as we developed and learned to move as infants. Re-introducing ourselves to our original movement plan is the foundation of *Original Strength* and it is the reason for its effectiveness. We are all "fearfully and wonderfully made" (Psalm 139:14) and some of the keys to unlocking better movement and health are already within us. They are there, in all of us, waiting to be re-discovered, and used to enhance our ability to live our lives to the fullest.

I was first introduced to Tim Anderson through Mr. John Brookfield, and shortly thereafter purchased a copy of his early work, ***Becoming Bulletproof***. The material was easy to understand and use. Within the pages of that first book, I learned of the "RESETS" I could use to re-store my movement capability. These RESETS, namely diaphragmatic breathing, neck nods, rolling, rocking, crawling and cross-crawling, seemed logical and were simple to put into practice. No steep learning curve, no complex combinations that required great skill or coordination.

I will admit when I first tried some of the RESETS, I smiled and giggled a bit, "Baby-Crawling? Are you kidding me?" The giggles became "Aha" moments more often as I regularly incorporated the RESETS into my daily schedule, in the mornings and before training. I noticed over the course of time, the range of motion I could attain when performing the RESETS improved and the movements themselves became more fluid and more intuitive. More importantly for me though, was the improvement in my "quality of life" activities, which at this point for me include playing alongside our children in whatever they are playing, meeting the physical requirements of my job, and lifting kettlebells.

Based on my personal experience with *Original Strength*, I believed incorporating it into our program would benefit our players' performance and ultimately, their well-being. So a couple of years ago, we invited Tim to visit our facility in order to introduce the fundamentals of *Original Strength* to my staff and me. My time with Tim added clarity to the concepts I had only read about up to that point, and refined my understanding of the RESETS as well as adding some variations we could use for our population, according to our specific needs. When he visited, Tim gave me a copy of the first edition of this book. Reading the information in *Original Strength* provided even greater insight, expanded my understanding of OS, and opened the door to a deeper exploration of our intended ability to move and play!

> *" I see the beauty in the simplicity of the Original Strength RESETS and the significant impact they can have on our amazingly intricate design.*

As of this writing, I continue to learn more about the anatomical and physiological principles that gird up the OS system, and as I do, I see the beauty in the simplicity of the *Original Strength* RESETS and the significant impact they can have on our amazingly intricate design. Over the past two years, we have incorporated the OS RESETS into programming for our players. Their initial reaction was similar to mine…giggles, but along with me, we press reset before most training opportunities and continue to explore and enjoy their impact on movement together.

In July of 2015, my family and I visited Tim and the OS Family in North Carolina to spend some quality time together, and also for Tim to teach our children the fundamentals of *Original Strength*. Everyone from young children to professional athletes can perform the RESETS in *Original Strength* and benefit from them; I have witnessed it first-hand with people in my life who are important to me. Please allow me to encourage you to read ***Pressing RESET, Original Strength Reloaded*** and consider making the RESETS the basis of your movement practice. Re-build your movement and live the amazing life intended for you!

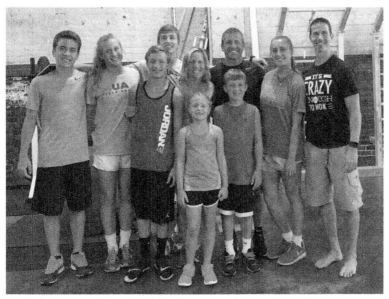

Tim Anderson & the Morton Family, July 2015

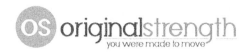

You Are Awesomely And Wonderfully Made

You are one of the most awesome creations the world has ever known. You are capable of almost anything because you were designed to be without limits. This is the truth.

In the beginning, you were created perfectly. When you were born, your brain had a movement template that was "hard wired" into it, and your body was a blank slate ready and willing to grow and express perfect strength and mobility. You spent your infant and toddler years learning how to move, building strength and completely integrating your whole body. You glued everything together: your nervous system, vestibular system (balance system), cardiovascular system, visual system, muscular system, proprioceptive system, digestive system—every system you have—you integrated and intertwined them all together. Your body became whole. It became one cohesive unit. You were one piece called a body, not one body of several parts, pieces and systems.

When you were a child, you experienced life through your design. Through learning how to move, you nourished and developed your brain and you built and developed your body, gaining strength by the day. As you developed, movement and strength became one and the same. You moved with the strength you developed, and the strength you developed helped you move. From the beginning, by the design of your original blueprint, you were meant to move with grace, fluidity, strength and power.

Every movement you made was a building block for the next movement you would take. You were developing and laying the perfect foundation for all physical, mental, and emotional expression. Then, one day, something happened, something changed. You no longer explored your world through movement. You stopped using your body and you became stagnant. You became "an adult" and you left behind your childish ways.

Now, that childhood has passed away, you intuitively know that something is wrong. You cannot move the way you wish you could. Nor do you feel as good as you know you should. In your recollection and imagination, you remember how strong you were when you were younger and you dream about things you wish you could do, but no longer can because of fear, pain, or lack of health. You toss out phrases like, "When you hit thirty, forty, fifty, etc… everything falls apart." Such phrases of defeat are only fact if you settle on them and believe them. However, they are never the truth. The truth is you can be strong and move well throughout your entire life. This is your design. As an adult, you still have the ability to experience life through your design.

> *" Just to be clear, when we are referring to "strength", we are talking about the ability to live life the way that you want to live it; to be able to move, think, work, play, love and laugh throughout your entire life, regardless of your age.*

Growing older should not mean becoming weak and frail. Your entire life was meant to be lived through strength. Just to be clear, when we are referring to "strength", we are talking about the ability to live life the way that you want to live it; to be able to move, think, work, play, love and laugh throughout your entire life, regardless of your age. We should be able to run, jump, climb and play without sustaining nagging injuries or acquiring other "movement issues." When we are 90 years old, we should still have a strong, healthy body that allows us to enjoy life.

Again, the body should not lose its strength just because it grows older. As we grow older, we should still be able to move around much like we did when we were teenagers, or the way we did when we were in our "glory years." We have to look through the deception of "age." Age should only represent a number, and nothing more. It should be an indication of the time a person has spent on earth. It should not be a death sentence. It should not represent usefulness, or ability. It is only a chronological reference point. A 70 year old can have every bit as much vitality and spring in their step as a 30 year old. Some do. Your body, all bodies, are designed to retain their strength, and even gain strength, regardless of your age.

Think about it. We really are awesomely and wonderfully made. What would be the point of growing older without vitality? We were meant to live, enjoy and make the most of this life. We were not meant to grow older only to lose our independence. That is not growing older, that is a slow conscious death. Eagles soar until the day they die. We were meant to do the same thing.

> *" Age should only represent a number, and nothing more.*

Becoming weak and frail happens to us when we spend our lives being static, when we allow stress and fears to consume us, when all we do is work and not play. Becoming fragile is a result of using our bodies, or not using our bodies rather, for something other than what they were intended. There is more to life than aches, pains, lethargy, apathy, obesity, unsteadiness, high blood pressure, diabetes, and heart disease. *You were not meant for any of these things!* Almost all of life's "issues" could, or can, be combated and defeated if we would regain our simple movement patterns and engage in them on a regular basis.

We were always intended to move, play and to engage in life. And we can. This is how we were designed to be.

How can you return to the Original You?

You simply do what you once did when you were a child: move according to your design. The same movement template which was placed in you as a child, the same original blueprint you were designed to carry out, is still inside of you right now. The same perfect strength and grace you were designed to have is still within you waiting to be expressed. You can regain the strength you once had, you can rise up with the strength you were meant to have, and reclaim the body that is rightfully yours.

By simply spending time on the floor and moving like a child, you can regain your *original strength*. Remembering how to breathe, controlling your head movements, rolling around on the floor, rocking back and forth, and even crawling around can re-establish wonderful reflexive connections throughout your entire body allowing you to express the strength and mobility that has always been yours to have.

We know this sounds crazy, but it is crazy enough to work!

If you want to have a resilient body, start moving like you did when you were a child. It is amazing what a difference this will make in your body. It is so amazing; it seems like a miracle. Engaging in "child-like" movements is the key to turning back the hands of time and reclaiming the body you were meant to have. We know this sounds too good to be true, but it is not too good to be true when you consider your body was designed to heal itself. Reversing the aging process through movement is simply the body's way of healing itself.

Life is meant to be enjoyed. If you really want to be able to enjoy your life, you need a healthy body. Being injured and being in pain should not be the norm or the status quo. It should not be a result of time simply passing us by! Even in our 90s, we should be able to go for a run without having knee pain. We should be able to pick up a suitcase without hurting our backs. We should be able to grab something out of the back seat of our car without tearing a rotator cuff. We should be resilient!

You are not supposed to be weak or fragile. Refuse to accept these conditions. Move and heal. No matter what the state of your body is right now, you can start where you are, regain your *original strength*, and return to the original You. Everything you need to become resilient and strong is already inside of your brain, waiting to be tapped into again.

Start moving like you did once upon a time. Learn how to PRESS RESET with your body and restore the body you were meant to have: A strong, flexible, powerful body capable of climbing any mountain or swimming any sea at **any age**. You are meant to grow old with strength and health, with grace and dignity. You do not have to be afraid of aging. You are meant to be able to wrestle with your grandkids and go for long walks with your friends and family. Growing older should be a wonderful process, not something to be dreaded and feared.

The majority of information in this book has been well researched and applied in the areas of learning disabilities, brain development and brain rehabilitation. We are extrapolating from these ideas used for building a healthy brain and applying this information, along with our own ideas, observations, and experiences, towards building a strong, healthy body. After all, brain health is not separate from the body's health. The brain and body are in union with one another. Improving one improves the other.

You are indeed awesomely and wonderfully made, always. Refuse to settle for anything less. Live your *original strength*.

The Steel Geezer

"I am what they call a high miler. I'm 68, but if my life had an odometer it would read in Roman Numerals. I qualify for two artificial knees and until I found Original Strength my rotator cuffs were rotator puffs. However, even if you combined these factors along with the lifelong back issues from heavy dead lifts and squats, one stroke and a 5th heart attack that literally killed me resulting in an Implantable Cardiac Defibrillator that looks like a can of sardines sticking out of my chest, everything was copacetic. OK, it was like, "Other than that Mrs. Lincoln, how was the theater?"

To be honest, I've faced death so many times the hairs on the back of my neck don't stand up any more. The death angel doesn't even bother showing up now; he figures it's just another false alarm. Besides, he knows I'm doing Original Strength.

How I discovered Tim Anderson and Original Strength could be summed up in just two words: divine intervention.

I have friends, family, medical records, a Sports Medicine Doctor, x-rays and a personal physician that will tell you the wonders that have taken place since I started practicing the Original Strength principles. I can do dips, chins, push-ups, squats, the whole enchilada—all pain free. Heck, I can even give myself a black eye with my knee if I get carried away doing my standing cross crawls, and I couldn't even kick the cat before.

Original Strength is principle based. I learned about principles 10 years ago from a gentleman who is a combat tactics, special ops instructor. My eyes were opened to the wondrous possibilities of a principle integrated life.

I learned that principles are immutable laws of universal reality. They are foundational, not mere techniques, tactics, procedures or opinions.

*They are applicable across the entire spectrum of human function; physically, mentally and spiritually. For this reason, there are no concerns regarding retention as these principles are already embedded in your human hard drive. You do not acquire their benefits, **they are yours by right**.*

The principles of Original Strength are simple, easy to integrate, and they work for anyone and everyone, enabling you to experience your inherent right to healing, resilience, and that special no-holds-barred life you are here to live.

Original Strength, endorsed by the Universe. Thanks Tim. "

- Freddie Mitchell, aka The Steel Geezer
Vancouver Island

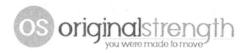

Life Starts With Movement

B abies develop perfectly through learning how to move. Even before a child sees the light of this world, he starts developing his brain and muscles inside his mother's womb through movement. Once a child is born, the reflexes and movement patterns already etched deep into his brain start building an amazing foundation of strength through movement exploration. In turn, this wonderful strength being developed through movement actually helps develop the brain and nervous system. The very movements creating a child's strength also further create his nervous system. In other words, our bodies and brain are developed through a cycle of movement. The more we move through our natural movement patterns, the more we develop our brain. The more we develop our brain, the more efficient we become at moving. The more efficient we become at moving, the better we move and the more we further develop our brain. This cycle can and should go on and on throughout our entire lives.

> " *Brain development and body development are not mutually exclusive events.*

In case any of the above paragraph was confusing, here is a summation:

When we were children, we learned to move through specific movement patterns etched deep inside our brains. As we moved using these patterns, we developed and strengthened both our bodies and our brains. Brain development and body development are not mutually exclusive events. They go hand in hand. As one develops, the other is nourished and developed. Learning to move and engaging in movement even develops who we are as individuals. In *The Well Balanced Child*, Ewout Van-Manen points out *"...physical movement is the basis for cognitive, social and emotional development."*[4] Let's look at the converse of Van-Manen's statement: A lack of cognitive, social, and emotional development can be traced back to a lack of movement.

The brain and the body nourish and develop each other. However, movement is the catalyst for this nourishment. Movement builds **everything** about you. Through movement

> *"...movement physically changes and improves your brain!*

we develop our "body map," our sense of self in space. This is called proprioception.[5] Our body is filled with sensors and proprioceptors in our skin, joints, tendons, and muscles that feed our brain with a sense of self every time we move and experience our environment. The more we move, the more we flood our brain with information from our proprioceptors about what our body is doing and where our body is at. This flood of information creates a good "body map", or "movement map" in our brains. The better our body map is, the better we move.

Not only does movement improve your proprioception, it actually physically changes and improves your brain! Physical activity develops brain tissue![6] Inside your brain, there are millions of nerve connections, or nerve networks. Movement improves the communication between these connections and actually cements new connections.[7] The better you move, the more efficient your brain becomes. **The more efficient your brain becomes, the better you move.**

Again, brain development and body development go hand in hand. It's a two-way street and movement is the vehicle. Movement is the key to every facet of our health. It shapes everything about us: Our brains, our bodies, who we are as people, our emotions, our hormones, even our mental health.[8]

Clearly, we were designed to move. Yet, most of us don't. Instead, we sit. So over time, we lose our movement patterns or we replace them with sitting. We slow our brain development. In some ways, our brain development regresses. This process is called neuronal fitness or neuronal pruning.[9] Just as movement can shape and develop our brains, not moving can also shape our brains. Simply put, for our brains to remain efficient they prune out the nerve connections we don't need or the ones we don't use often. The neural connections in the brain are much like the movement patterns in the body: Use it or lose it.

We live in a world filled with technological innovations and conveniences. We have computers, cars, and the Internet. There is no need for us to get up and move. If we want to go shopping, we only have to jump online and push a button or two. We don't even have to get out and go to the mall anymore! Every year we grow further and further away from physical bodies capable of anything and towards bodies capable of being paper weights. We are wonderfully made, yet we don't allow ourselves to participate in the wonder for which we were created. Instead of moving anywhere and everywhere, most of us spend our time going nowhere. We occupy the same square footage of a chair for hours and hours every day. Many kids today are not even learning how to run, how to skip, or how to climb. We are moving further and further away from what we were made for: movement. Movement is life, and life is movement!

In our civilized world, there are some things we cannot change. Kids have to go to school and adults have to go to work. In today's world we are going to spend a lot of time sitting. However, that doesn't mean we can't learn to minimize the time we spend sitting, and it doesn't mean we can't keep our bodies fit and capable of doing anything. We can learn to move deliberately and consistently, even if all we do is participate in small "movement snacks" throughout the day. Through consistent engagement, we can regain our movement patterns and rid ourselves of our movement limitations. We can rebuild our solid foundation of strength and movement, our *original strength*!

This is so important: In our lifetimes, we are not meant to have only a "season" of health. The body is far too amazing for such a season. Even if there was a season of health, seasons repeat themselves. Springtime comes around every year. New growth and repair always come back around. The body is designed to heal and repair itself. The "season" of restoration and repair starts with moving. It also ends when moving stops.

To live in a season of health, all we have to do is learn how to move the way we once did. To do this, we need only look at how children grow and develop. Babies move to live. They build a foundation of strength through reflexes and movement patterns deeply rooted inside their brains. From these reflexes and movement patterns, they learn to move in all possible combinations of movements and in all planes of motion. Their movement exploration builds strong, healthy, resilient bodies, and brains. Bodies meant to last a lifetime.

The simple, childish movements you once made can return the feeling of youth you once had. One of the greatest joys we receive when teaching at an *Original Strength* workshop is witnessing people rediscover movements, or abilities, they imagined were lost forever. At an *Original Strength* workshop in Chicago, we watched a 75 year young man rediscover he could squat all the way down, "butt to calves", like he could when he was a young man. Minutes before this discovery, he was only able to squat about one-fourth of the way down, not really low enough to even comfortably sit into a chair. Can you imagine the hope and the possibilities that emerged for this gentleman? He was probably resigned to the "fact" that he could not squat all the way down to the ground—he hadn't done it in years. Yet, after 3 minutes of BREATHING the way he was designed to, his range of motion was restored to him.

The season of restoration is now.

A Season of Restoration

"I just completed reading your book. I have a history of back issues and dislocation of my Sacroiliac joint on the right side. I have managed these inconveniences with a consistent combination of yoga, running, strength training, seriously limiting time spent sitting, and PT when needed. Having seen few, if any, positive outcomes with surgical or pain medication intervention, I have avoided those avenues.

I recently have experienced rather uncomfortable levels of pain related to the sacral issue. After reading the cross-crawl, crawling, rocking and rolling instructions, I went to my mat and did all of these. Let me just say, the pain relief is miraculous! I am moving more fluidly and with no pain or stiffness after sitting. This is after one short session.

This technique seems to have reset the pelvis better than the bridge exercise prescribed by my physical therapist. What an amazing difference. I had a pain free night of sleep for the first time in many months. I cannot tell you how excited I am!"

My Best Wishes,
Sharon Steedly

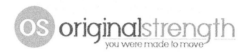

The X is in You

The road, or the map, to regaining our *original strength* revolves around the center of the X. The X is you. And the center of your X, and you, is your midsection, or your core. Having a reflexively strong and solid center is the key to regaining your *original strength*. Without a solid center, you will never be able to be as strong as you should be.

> **"Having a reflexively strong and solid center is the key to regaining your original strength.**

Please note, a reflexively strong center is not something you can get from doing traditional abdominal exercises. It is built by engaging in your original movement patterns. These developmental movement patterns stimulate, sharpen and cement your reflexes. Truly, a solid center is developed through global input from the entire body. It's the simplest of things, really, that contribute to make one resilient. Diaphragmatic breathing, engaging in developmental movement patterns, controlling the movements of the head, stimulating the skin, even the way we think—all of these, and more, contribute to building a powerful center, thus producing a powerful body.

We are fully integrated. Everything about you works together to make your whole body powerful and strong. If you were to remove any one facet of your body, like wearing thick soled shoes all of your life so that your feet could never feel the ground, or if you tried to isolate one of your body's systems from another, you would weaken your entire body. A child develops an amazingly strong body by exploration and fully integrating movement with his or her senses and systems. An adult can do the same thing. You can restore your strong center, you can rebuild your X, by engaging in and exploring the same movements you did as a developing child.

Again, you are the X. That is, your body is an X. Not only are you shaped like one big X, but your entire body is made up of a series of Xs. Just look at an anatomy chart of muscles and notice how the muscles and tendons lie in relationship to one another. Even your DNA is in the shape of a double helix, a spiraling X. The body is literally a series of connected Xs from head to toe.

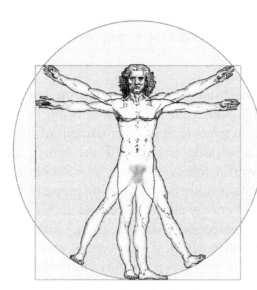

Can you see the X?

This is the drawing that actually inspired this chapter.

Draw a couple of diameter lines through any part of the circle. They cross at the man's navel. His navel is in the absolute center of the circle. The center is the secret to strength.

Leonardo da Vinci—Vitruvian Man
Public Domain Image

You also move in an "X-like" fashion. You are a contra-lateral moving being. At least you should be. When you walk, your left arm should match the swing of your right leg, and your right arm should match the swing of your left leg. Every step you take should be a fluid, coordinated motion bringing your opposite shoulders towards your opposite hips.

Even the way your nervous system is wired to move your body is played out in an "X-like" fashion. The right side of your brain controls the left side of your body and the left side of your brain controls the right side of your body. Again, everything about you is an X.

Is the Force Strong Within You?

In order for you to be as strong and resilient as you were meant to be, the center of your X must be knit together properly; much like a tightly woven Chinese finger trap. The center of your X, your core, is where the forces you generate from movement cross over from one side of your body to the other. These forces cross through your center from left to right, right to left, bottom to top, and top to bottom. The more "connected" your X is, the more efficient the forces can cross over. You are made to be efficient and powerful.

Think of your center as the area from your pelvic floor, the bottom of your bottom, to your armpits, with your belly button being in the dead center. However you think of the core, it is the crossroads of force production. When everything is working as it should, the core is the crossroads of efficient and powerful forces—the key to a strong and resilient body.[10] When things in the core are not functioning properly, the core can become the crossroads of energy chaos; forces end up going in areas they shouldn't go, creating unnecessary stresses, energy leakages, and movement dysfunctions. In other words, if your center, your core, is not functioning properly, you will not be as powerful or as resilient as you were meant to be, and you may be at a higher risk of injury, as well as a myriad of other issues like poor digestion, unbalanced hormones, sluggish metabolism and so on.

Baseballs are Durable

In order to understand the importance of having a solid center, it may help to look at the difference between baseballs and whiffle balls. A baseball is pretty durable. Babe Ruth could hit a 300-plus yard home-run with the same baseball 100 times. As long as he never lost the baseball, he would be able to hit that same ball over and over again. Why? Because a baseball is solid. It has a solid center. The forces coming from Babe's powerful swing travel through the center of the ball and the ball travels outside the park. After a while, the stitching may start to give way, and the cover may start to unravel, but the ball is still a ball and Babe could still play with it. The baseball is very resilient. Because it is solid, it can absorb and transfer large amounts of energy, repeatedly, without becoming damaged.

Whiffle balls, on the other hand, are not so durable. Babe Ruth could hit a whiffle ball and it may only travel as far as second base. It would not even come close to making it outside of the ball park. And, if he were lucky, The Babe may be able to get one more hit out of the whiffle ball before it cracked or split. Why? Whiffle balls are hollow, they are empty. The forces coming from Babe's powerful swing would travel around the shell of the whiffle ball. These forces would ultimately be too great for the shell to remain intact, causing it to split. Whiffle balls are pretty fragile when it comes to absorbing and transferring energy. They can survive the hits of small children, but they can't withstand the powerful blows of an adult.

We were created to be more like the baseball, not the whiffle ball. The human body needs to have a solid center to effectively transfer all the forces it generates and all the other forces life throws at it (think of life as the baseball bat.)

Did you know that the human body produces two times it's weight in force when you walk, in every single step you take? If you weighed only 100 pounds and you walked 1000 steps, you would be producing 200 pounds of force with every step you made. When you run, you generate six to eight times your weight in force. When you sprint, you generate ten to twelve times your weight! For a 100 pound person, that would be 1000 pounds of force generated with every single step made in a 100 meter dash! How many people do you know who only weigh 100 pounds?

Can you see why it is so important for your X to have a solid center? Those powerful forces we generate and encounter need to travel efficiently and appropriately through our bodies. If we have a "hollow" center, if our X is not properly tied together, then we could become quite fragile, like the whiffle ball.

The baseball and whiffle ball analogy is perhaps an overly simplistic explanation, but hopefully it paints an idea of the importance of needing a solid center to be and stay durable. Your body was created to last and withstand the ravages of time and life. You are even meant to be more durable than a baseball!

You Are Fully Integrated

Remember, your body is fully integrated. Your X is knit together by everything about you. Your head movement is tied to your core.[11] Your grip is tied to your core. Your feet are tied to your core. Your skin is tied to your core. Your emotions are even tied to your core. Your core is tied to **EVERYTHING**. Your entire body is interconnected and this interconnection is what solidifies your center. Isn't this fascinating? Nothing about you is isolated from any part of you. **Everything about you is integrated.** Your body was created to be in perfect union with itself.

Unfortunately, people are really good at not honoring their design. We create conveniences in life that allow us to be comfortable so we don't have to move. Things like chairs, rearview mirrors, computers, remote controls (children!), etc. We have become really good at not moving our heads or our bodies. We have become masters of disintegration. In return, we lose some of our movement patterns, we stagnate our vestibular system (we dull or lose our balance), we lose our reflexively stable core, and we become broken. We lose these things not simply because we do not use them, but because we do not need them with our current lifestyles.

Fortunately, we can knit our centers back together again, and regain our *original strength*. If we really want to become physically resilient and strong, we need to do what babies do: Build our strength and mobility through movement.

Babies actually develop their strength and resiliency through specific movements we call "RESETS." These "RESETS" are just that, a reset. When we engage in these RESETS, strength is reborn.

Connecting The X

"I've gotten tremendous results when I put crawling into serious practice. Not only have I increased my strength, endurance and flexibility but I think I have found the most important thing: freedom. If you are familiar with some Systema Martial Arts practitioners (if not check on youtube), you can see that they are moving with grace and power. I discovered this grace and power from doing the OS RESETS, not only from crawling. By the way, Systema is based on breathing, another wonderful concept from OS.

Now, I am not an emotional slave to the other tools and training methods. Now, everything has become the tool! A rock, table, stairs, a bench, the floor, I can use and train with everything! This is freedom. I can move my body in all positions and directions with grace and I don't worry about injuries. I have true resilience and freedom. So crawling is much more than a strength and conditioning tool for me. I will always recommend the OS RESETS to people around me, because I know the power behind those 'silly' moves. I am not a believer anymore, I just know as I have experienced this to be true in my life. Even if I do get an injury, I have confidence because I know the OS RESETS."

–Łukasz (Luke)
Poland

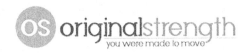

Pressing RESET

Have you ever been frustrated with your computer or your "smart" phone because it froze up on you or it just didn't seem to be working properly? What did you do? More than likely, you rebooted it. Usually, rebooting our technological devices, seems to magically return them to proper working order. When we reboot our devices, the operating system gets refreshed and all is well with our world.

What if you could reboot your body? What if you were not able to move the way you know you should be able to move, or you weren't as strong as you know you should be? What if you could simply press a reset button and reboot your body's operating system?

> **"Reflexive control is the foundation of our movement expression.**

You can!

Engaging in the same developmental movements you made as a child, the movements preprogrammed into your operating system, whether you did them as a child or not, is like pressing a reset button on your body. In fact, this book is about five developmental movements, and their variations, we call *RESETS*. Engaging in any one, or all, of these movements, *RESETS* our operating systems and our bodies respond by functioning in proper working order.

How does this happen? "Pressing reset" refreshes the nervous system and it also restores the proper reflexive connections throughout the body, returning your *reflexive control*.

Reflexive control is the foundation of our movement expression. It is the combination, or union rather, of reflexive stability, reflexive mobility and reflexive strength. The more reflexive control we have, the more we are able to express movement and participate in all the wonderful hobbies and skills we want to perform in life: A ballerina cannot perform ballet without reflexive control. When we do not have all of our reflexive strength, stability, or mobility, we do not have our full reflexive control and we cannot fully express all the mobility, strength, power, speed and fluidity that we were designed to express.

> " *The truth is, strength, stability and mobility are all components of the same thing: movement, or the control of movement.*

As the body is often viewed in separate parts, mobility is also viewed as a separate quality from stability or strength. Mobility was never meant to be segregated from stability or strength. That is certainly not how the body develops or operates. The truth is, strength, stability and mobility are all components of the same thing: movement, or the control of movement.

For example, when a child learns how to lift its very large head, it is building stability, strength, AND mobility. Yes, babies are born mobile, but they are like rag dolls. They cannot control their mobility. It is only

36

when they build the strength and stability to move and hold their heads on the horizon that they also develop the *control* of their mobility. If any one of these qualities is lacking, they are all lacking. They were all designed to be built together, in unison with one another.

They are also designed to operate together, in unison. For example, if a man lacks the mobility to be able to touch his toes, more than likely it is because he lacks the reflexive stability in his core to stabilize his spine. The brain is smart. If the body's stabilizers, the muscles that stabilize joints, are not working properly, the brain turns prime movers, the muscles that move joints, into stabilizers. When prime movers become stabilizers, they can no longer move the body the way they were intended and the mobility of the body is limited. When mobility is limited, strength is limited. Thus the body cannot optimally express its full potential for strength, mobility or stability because the overall movement expression—*reflexive control*—is limited.

When we Press RESET and engage our original operating system, we begin to restore and regain our reflexive control, our foundation—we restore our reflexive strength, mobility and stability. They are all parts of the same expression and they are all controlled by our reflexes. This is the foundation our strength, health and resiliency are built upon. In order to become as healthy and resilient as possible, we have to own our reflexive control. We do this by Pressing Reset often and *consistently* in order to deepen our "roots" and establish a foundation of reflexive control constantly reinforced and nurtured throughout the rest of our lifespan.

To be extremely honest, we cannot fully understand how Pressing RESET works. Science is still discovering how amazing the body is and how what "we" thought we knew about the body, "we" don't really know. Not too long ago, many scientist *knew* once the brain lost neural connections, they were lost forever. But now scientists know that the brain is "plastic." No, the brain is not made out of petroleum byproducts, but it is "plastic" in that it is capable of change. This is called neuroplasticity. This is such great news! Your brain is capable of constant change and growth moment by moment.

Even though we cannot scientifically explain how Pressing RESET works, we can however, tell you it does indeed work. We don't have to understand how our computers are programmed to be able to reboot them. We still know how to reboot them and restore them to their default settings when they don't seem to be working properly.

The OS Big Five

Original Strength consists of five developmental movement patterns we call RESETS. Engaging in these movements, pressing reset, refreshes the central nervous system, it creates efficient neural pathways in both the brain and the body, and it restores and "sharpens" reflexive neuromuscular connections. Consistently engaging in these movements embeds these neural connections so they WILL NOT go away. The result of having a brain and body full of efficient, "sharp" neural connections, is having a body fully capable of expressing its original design; in both movement as well as thought. This is how we can restore our *original strength!*

Here are the OS Big Five:

1. Diaphragmatic breathing
2. Head Control, specifically head nods
3. Rolling
4. Rocking
5. Crawling/Cross-crawling/Gait patterns

In the chapters that follow, we shall explore the details of each of these RESETS. But before we do that, let's take a look at the ONLY rules inside of *Original Strength*. We emphasize the word "only" here because when it comes to pressing reset, there is no algorithm! Every person has a different history wrapped up inside of their body and any reset can be the reset they need. The RESETS will be presented in this book in the child developmental sequence, but they need not be applied in this sequence to be effective. There is no correct order for pressing reset. You don't have to pass GO before you can collect $200. A reset button is a reset button. There is no algorithm and there are no rules. Well, there are no "rules," but there are three principles:

The Three Principles of the OS Big Five

There are only three principles we follow when it comes to pressing reset. These three principles were all addressed when you were a developing child, and they are addressed when we engage in the five movements that we call RESETS:

1. You must breathe properly, with your diaphragm
2. You must activate your vestibular system—you have to move your head.
3. You must cross midline with your limbs and/or engage in your contra-lateral movement patterns (like crawling or walking).

If you follow these three simple principles, you can return to your original design and become as strong and healthy as you could ever want to be, as you were meant to be.

The Hope in Movement

"I was diagnosed with ALS five years ago. It's a disease that robs the muscles of their motor neurons; resulting in limited movement. Since my personal goal was to keep my body active and moving for as long as possible, I had to learn "how" to move all over again—from the ground up! Incorporating the Original Strength RESETS into my daily exercise has helped me both regain and retain my body's fundamental movement patterns. In fact, all the Original Strength information and exercises are informative and helpful. I learned how to maintain my core strength, joint mobility, sense of balance and have a positive attitude. Five years after my diagnosis, I am moving on!"

–Dagmar Munn
Arizona

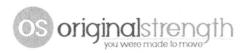

The Breath of Life

Breathing properly is vital to regaining your original strength. If you are not breathing properly, learning how to breathe could be the most important concept in this entire book. Breathing is perhaps the most overlooked, undervalued, and most critical reflex you possess.

When a child is born, the first real reflex and movement they engage in is breathing. Babies breathe correctly right from the start: They use their diaphragms. Babies don't breathe high up in their chest like most adults do. Instead, they pull air down deep into their lungs with their diaphragm. Breathing with the diaphragm is how children first start strengthening the center of their X. Yes, breathing is not simply exchanging oxygen and carbon dioxide. It is also strength training. When a child is breathing, they are not merely just "breathing", they are strength training.

" Breathing is perhaps the most overlooked, undervalued, and most critical reflex you possess.

For various reasons, adults unlearn, or retrain, this natural breathing reflex. Many adults trade deep "belly breathing" (diaphragmatic breathing) for shallow "chest breathing." In doing so, they weaken their core, the center of their X.

If this is you, if you are a chest breather, relearning and regaining your natural way of breathing can be the greatest step you ever take towards regaining your *original strength.* In fact, it may be impossible to unlock your full strength and health potential without breathing properly. All your attempts to becoming healthy and resilient will be stacked up on a faulty breathing pattern—a faulty foundation, a pattern that will only strengthen weakness and stress.

Just in case you don't remember, when you were born, you were a diaphragmatic breather, or a "belly breather." You were born this way for a reason. Just watch any newborn baby. You will see their little bellies rise up and down when they breathe. They are taking full advantage of their lung volume by effortlessly breathing with their diaphragm (let's call it the "breathing muscle"). The diaphragm pulls a vacuum in the lungs allowing them to fill themselves full of life-giving air. Diaphragmatic breathing also massages the internal organs thus aiding in digestion. And, perhaps most surprisingly, the diaphragm works together with the pelvic floor and the other muscles in your center to help create a reflexively stable, strong core.

> **" Your diaphragm is like the "captain" of your inner core musculature**

Your diaphragm is like the "captain" of your inner core musculature, the center of your center. When you breathe with the diaphragm, your diaphragm works in unison with these inner core muscles providing reflexive stability and protection for your spine. It may help to imagine that the diaphragm and the pelvic floor both work together to form a "cylinder of strength" in your center. The more solid your center is, the more strength, power, speed, and resilience you will possess.

Again, you were born breathing with your diaphragm. Some people, *most people*, end up retraining how they breathe by using their accessory breathing muscles, or the muscles in their rib cage, neck and shoulders. The accessory breathing muscles are the muscles a baby uses to breathe when his breathing is compromised and he is in distress. When babies use these muscles to breathe, they are usually sick and may need emergency medical attention. It may help to think of these accessory breathing muscles as *emergency breathing muscles*.

For some reason, whether it is due to stressful lives, or because people are trying to hide their guts, they become "chest breathers." They use their emergency breathing muscles to breathe; twenty-four hours a day, seven days a week.

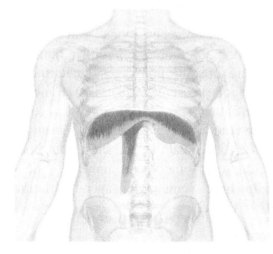

This is what the diaphragm looks like. It is a *muscle*. It is this muscle that truly makes you resilient.

And like most muscles, the diaphragm can be trained. It can grow stronger and efficient with use!

From Tim:

I am fairly certain I know exactly when I started using my emergency breathing muscles. It was when I was in middle school. I was a very scrawny kid, and as you probably know, middle school can be a harsh world for insecure teenagers. I didn't want to get picked on, beat up, or singled out, so I started sucking in my gut and puffing out my chest. I was trying to look much bigger than I was. It didn't work! I still got picked on, and I became a chest breather. The stress of middle school and the fear of being the weakest one in the herd was strong enough to make me override my natural breathing pattern. It can start as simple as that for anyone. There is an upside down lesson here: the desire to simply look stronger can actually make you weaker.

We do have accessory respiratory muscles for a reason, they are, our emergency breathing muscles. They are reserved for emergencies or times of extreme stress. We shouldn't need to use these breathing muscles all the time. They are our startle, or fight or flight breathing muscles. Breathing with these emergency breathing muscles can cause a myriad of unwanted issues throughout the body.

Danger, Danger!

Constantly living and breathing in "emergency mode" can cause a forward head carriage, neck pain, poor thoracic mobility, hunched forward posture, early fatigue when exercising, poor digestion, hormonal imbalances, inflammation, high blood pressure, cardiac issues, mental inabilities to cope with stress, and if that were not enough, it can cause a loss of reflexive stability in the core muscles of the body. If you are always breathing with your emergency breathing muscles, your body is always in stress mode, which is a very inefficient, unhealthy mode to be stuck in for a long period of time. Some people spend a lifetime breathing like this. Are you one of them?

The good news is if we can change our breathing pattern *for the bad*, then we can also retrain our breathing pattern and change it back *for the good*. Breathing is a natural subconscious reflex (like all reflexes). However, breathing can also be controlled and trained consciously.

In the *Original Strength* workshops, we introduce crocodile breathing as one way to relearn how to diaphragmatically breathe. In crocodile breathing, you lay on your belly and rest your forehead on the back of your hands. While inhaling through your nose, keep your tongue on the roof of your mouth and try to breathe deep down into your belly. If you do this correctly, your belly will push against the floor and cause your lower back to rise up. The sides of your belly will also expand and get wider, just like a crocodile! This can be a very effective way to retrain yourself how to become a belly breather. It is not the only way however.

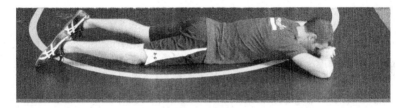

There are many ways in which one can practice belly breathing. We cover a series of breathing "regressions" in our workshops that help many people rediscover the magic of breathing and its correlation to better movement and performance.

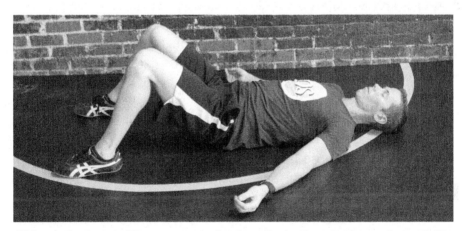

This particular position seems to be favorite in the group sessions at the Original Strength Institute. Look, it even puts Tim to sleep...

Perhaps the most effective way to remember how to breathe is to just spend time on the floor like a child and deliberately try to breathe deep into your belly while you explore different positions. You may need to rest your hands on your belly to increase awareness of your desired target, or imagine you are trying to breathe all the way down to the bottom of your feet to encourage deep breaths. It doesn't matter *how you do it*, as long as you *can do it*—effortlessly, in any position.

Hold Your Tongue But Don't Hold Your Breath

While we are on the subject of breathing, we need to mention the tongue. Believe it or not, where you keep your tongue matters. In fact, it may be a critical detail to your overall health. Your tongue is designed to rest against the roof of your mouth, behind your front teeth. This is the "home position" for your tongue, and this is also a reset button. We often call this position, or this action, the *reset within the RESETS*.

Placing the tongue on the roof of the mouth encourages nasal breathing. Nasal breathing encourages diaphragmatic breathing. You can breathe diaphragmatically through your mouth, but you are designed to naturally breathe through your nose. (This is how we are able to smell things!) Please understand, breathing through the nasal passages is *optimal*, but some people may not be able to due to having restricted nasal passages because of issues like a broken nose, a deviated septum, or other restrictions.

If, however, you are able to breathe through your nasal passages, you should make an effort to do so as there are numerous benefits to doing so. Again, one of those benefits is it encourages the diaphragm to do its job. Another benefit of breathing through the nose is it can make you stronger. Nasal passages are smaller than the opening of the mouth. Breathing in through these smaller, narrow passages actually helps create more inter-abdominal pressure between your diaphragm and your pelvic floor. This increased inter-abdominal pressure helps you become stronger and more resilient by creating a "muscle girdle" through and around your center. In our baseball versus whiffle ball analogy, this is like upgrading the baseball to a better, even more resilient model. This higher pressurized "muscle girdle" is built and maintained through the reflexive action of diaphragmatic breathing through the nasal passages. Breathing through the nasal passages usually happens when we shut our mouths and keep our tongues in the "home position."

Strength Starts Here

Truly, breathing with your diaphragm is the beginning of strength. This is how you first started tying your X together. Using your diaphragm as it was intended can mean the difference between being durable like the baseball, or being fragile like the whiffle ball.

" *breathing with your diaphragm is the beginning of strength*

Relearning how to breathe properly can also unlock a whole host of health benefits. When a person is breathing properly, they are not in "emergency mode," but rather they are in "rest and digest mode", or "peace mode." Diaphragmatic breathers have more peace. Their bodies, and their minds, are able to rest. Being at rest allows one to cope with life's stressors. It allows one to digest their food properly, keeping a healthy metabolism, and it allows one to sleep better. The mind and the body need to be able to rest. Rest and sound sleep are restorative.

Ponder with me. If you are subconsciously breathing with your emergency breathing muscles during the day when you are awake, how are you breathing at night when you are asleep? Just something to ponder...

Real strength comes from being able to live in a state of peace. Where the mind leads, the body will follow. If your thoughts are stressful and chaotic, your body will also reflect stress and chaos in your movements. If your thoughts are calm and fluid, your body will reflect your mind with calm and fluid movements. Life is not supposed to be a constant emergency. Even if it was, we were created to overcome and mitigate the emergency through calm, steady strength—through breath! Simply put, you can survive, but you were made to thrive.

It is vitally important you breathe the way you were designed to breathe. If you do not, you will never operate in the full capacity of your design. If this were the only thing you learned how to do from this book, it alone, would be enough to change your life for the better. Your *original strength*, the foundation of you, starts with a breath. You must use your diaphragm. Please do not dismiss this simple truth.

Breathe:

- Assume the desired position above.
- Keep your mouth closed.
- Place (rest) your tongue on the roof of your mouth. (If you're not sure exactly where this position is or how it should feel, just swallow, and your tongue will go there automatically.)
- Breathe in and out through your nose.
- Pull air deep down into your belly.
- Become strong!

Take A Breath

"I have a client that had a chronic hip flexor problem and couldn't even pry himself with a crowbar into a squat. Once his breathing pattern changed from chest breathing to diaphragm breathing, he can now hang out in a rock bottom squat for a time. This was the first time his pain went away in 5 years since a mountain bike accident which triggered his dysfunction."

Trevor Trebbien
Oregon

"Diaphragmatic breathing is great for movement, but also has many other applications. In my work with students in the military, it's taught as 'tactical breathing'. We use it in teaching marksmanship. Tactical breathing can be used to slow the heart rate in order to make a precise long distance shot, or it can help with getting accurate hits with a handgun.

We also teach students to use it to help control stress in many situations. I've had students become successful using it during some of our more stressful meeting and negotiation scenarios to calm themselves as things get tense. An example of how diaphragmatic breathing could be helpful in a stressful environment would be if you were standing, you might ask to have a seat. During that short amount of time you move to sit down, if you 'set your breathing' it will help you gain some clarity and you can refocus, mitigating your stress.

Just as with Original Strength, it may seem to be a small part of the process...but in reality it's a vital root to the process. We believe in using diaphragmatic breathing in situations that could be life or death, national strategic-level success or failure, or just keeping a calm head."

Chad Faulkner
US Army

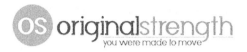

You Have To Use Your Head

The next reset we will discuss involves learning how to use your head. Learning how to move the head, developing head control, is how a child starts adding to the layer of strength created by breathing with the diaphragm. For children, as well as for adults, mastering head control is essential to balance, posture, and coordination.[12] Another way to say this is mastering head control is essential for strength.

The Vestibular System

> *"mastering head control is essential for strength*

The reason head control is so important to your overall strength and health is because your vestibular system (your balance system) lives in your head, right behind your ears. The vestibular system is made up of highly sensitive organs called the utricle, saccule, and semicircular canals.[13] Without getting too scientific, they are like having your own internal gyroscopes inside your head. These organs are filled with tiny hairs and a gel-like substance. When your head moves, the liquid substance moves these tiny hairs and sends information to your brain. Your gyroscopes work to give you equilibrium and balance.[14] Their job is to keep your head level with the horizon.

You have two of these in your head. One behind each ear. These tiny little gyroscopes are what make you who you are.

A healthy vestibular system is necessary for a healthy, strong body. In fact, total health cannot exist separate from a healthy vestibular system. The vestibular system is perhaps the most important sensory system you have. Everything about you is shaped by how your vestibular system functions: Your sense of self, your reality, your balance, your posture, your ability to hold your head up and maintain your gaze with the horizon, your ability to learn, your experiences, everything.[15]

You can function without other sensory systems and lead a somewhat "normal" life. For instance, a blind man can learn to be independent and get around almost as well as people who have sight. But a person with a damaged vestibular system may not be able to have a "normal" life. Just ask anyone who has ever had vertigo and they will tell you how important a healthy vestibular system is for feeling "normal" and healthy.

VESTIBULAR SYSTEM

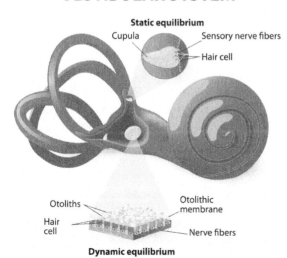

You have two of these in your head. One behind each ear. These tiny little gyroscopes are what make you who you are.

51

One of the reasons we think the vestibular system is one of, if not THE, most important sensory system you have is because it is the first sensory system to begin developing in the fetus, inside the mother's womb. It begins developing about 21 days after conception,[16] and is fully developed about 5 months after conception.[17] Four months before a child is born he has a functioning vestibular system. Every movement the mother makes provides stimulation to the functioning vestibular system. This stimulation helps develop the child's brain and nervous system.

Once the child is born, the new world of gravity and all the challenges it brings begin to further stimulate the vestibular system. All of this stimulation and activation created by gravity and the child's own movements shape the nervous system and build the child into the person he will become. Movement shapes the brain.

The vestibular system is also extremely important because it is also the foundation all other sensory systems are built upon or routed through. In fact, all the systems in the body and all the information received by the body are routed through the vestibular system.[18] Your vestibular system is the hub for all the information that goes into your brain. It is this information, in combination with the information generated by the vestibular system itself, that feeds and nourishes your brain and creates who you are.

This includes the information provided by your proprioceptive system, or your inner sense of self. The proprioceptive system is the collection of information about what your body is doing and what is going on around your body. It is intimately tied to your vestibular system.[19] Together, they form your body map, or your movement map. The better your movement map is, the better you move.

Your visual system is also tied to your vestibular system. Ninety percent of the cells in your visual system respond to vestibular information.[20] Your autonomic nervous system (the system that controls the things you don't consciously control like your heart rate, respiratory rate, your digestion, perspiration, arousal, etc.) is tied to your vestibular system.[21] The vestibular system is also connected to every single muscle in your body, especially the core and neck muscles![22] Even your emotions can be affected by your vestibular system.[23] Everything about you is connected to your vestibular system.

Therefore, a healthy vestibular system is crucial to having a healthy body. How do you build a healthy vestibular system? Well, your vestibular system is designed to

> " *a healthy vestibular system is crucial to having a healthy body*

detect movement and receive information. If you feed that design, you can improve its function. When you were a child, you fed the design. Today as an adult, you can build a healthy vestibular system the same way: move! The more you move, the more you stimulate your vestibular system. The more you stimulate your vestibular system, the more neural connections you make in your brain and your body. You can literally move your way to having a healthier vestibular system, thus having a healthier, stronger, more resilient body.

It has even been shown that children who receive regular vestibular stimulation show advanced development in motor skills.[24] Remember, all your muscles are tied to your vestibular system. If you continually stimulate your vestibular system, you are essentially stimulating all of the muscles in your body, especially your core and neck muscles. Isn't that awesome? Not only that, but the more you stimulate and strengthen your vestibular system, the more you strengthen, or solidify, the health of all of your body's other systems. You are completely integrated. Improving any part of you improves the whole of you. Your vestibular system is not merely any part of you. It is a foundational part of you, if not THE foundational part of you. You CANNOT function properly without it.

If movement improves the vestibular system and heals the body, then not moving does just the opposite. When you don't move, you are not stimulating the vestibular system. In other words, you are not stimulating your brain, your nervous system, or your muscular system. Think of it this way, everything about the body follows the rule, "use it or lose it." The vestibular system is no different. If you do not train one of your most important senses or systems, it will begin to deteriorate much like your calculus skills slipped away after your graduated college.

It is interesting to note in the book,*The Well Balanced Child*, Sally Goddard Blythe points out one of the first signs of brain deterioration is when balance starts to deteriorate.[25] Why would brain deterioration and balance deterioration be linked together like this? Because your balance system (vestibular system) is the system that keeps your brain healthy. If you see someone who displays good balance and movement, you see someone with a healthy brain. How is your balance? Do you move with grace? Do you control your movements? Do you balance?

Heads are Heavy

When you were a child, you built a healthy vestibular system, brain and body by waging war against gravity. And it was a war, and you were at a disadvantage. Why? Because your head was insanely large compared to the rest of your tiny body. An infant's head weighs about 33% as much as their entire body weighs and it is about 25% as big as their entire body. Therefore, gravity has the advantage.

Learning how to move the head is where the layers of strength start to become solidified. As a baby, you persistently, consistently labored to move your head around. Due to your righting reflex, the reflex designed to keep your head level with the horizon, you learned how to pick your head up, hold it up, then keep it up. This is an amazing feat of strength when you think about it. Have you seen how tiny a baby's neck is? Can you imagine how weak your neck would seem if today your head weighed 33% as much as your body? If you only weighed 100 pounds, that would be like having a 33 pound head! The adult head weighs about ten to 12 pounds! Babies are ridiculously strong.

Remember, your vestibular system is connected to every single muscle in your body, especially the core musculature of the abdominals and back. It is these muscles that first work together to move the head.[26] Moving the neck and head is tied to your core musculature. When a child picks up his gargantuan sized head while lying on the floor, he is developing his core, the center of his X, and he is becoming amazingly strong.

From Tim:

As stated above, mastering head control is essential for obtaining strength. When a child learns to control his head, he owns the strength that adults would envy. I once watched Geoff's baby boy, Michael, hold his head up for over 5 minutes while lying on the floor. He was on his belly, and the only thing touching the floor was his belly! His head was held up high to see the world and his arms and legs were off the ground. He was doing a "back bridge" while pivoting around in circles on his belly. This fascinated me. So, when I was home alone, I tried it. I managed to make it through a brutal 5 minutes. I was shaking after one minute. For two whole days, may entire posterior side (my back side) was extremely sore. Even walking hurt. I only did that for 5 minutes, period. Little Michael did it for 5 minutes at a time throughout the entire day. Sure, my limbs were much longer than Michael's, but his head was much larger and heavier than mine, relatively.

Babies develop impressive strength. Adults should have impressive strength, too. But, that is not typically the case as most adults really don't move their heads too often. If every muscle in the body is connected to the vestibular system, and movement of the head affects every muscle in the body, then not moving the head also affects every muscle in the body. Not moving the head is like not stimulating all the muscles of the body. When muscles are not stimulated, they atrophy. When neural connections are not used, they get pruned, or they fade away. This is where weakness moves into the body.

Head Nods—The Controversial Reset

When we wrote the first edition back in 2013, there was a growing trend in the fitness industry towards making the simple complicated—especially when it came to the neck. In fact, some of the recommendations were based on the faulty interpretations of the body's function overall, including the design of the neck, its relation to the rest of the body, and its amazing integration with the body's reflexes.

Some were vocal proponents of "packing the neck"—which is a combination of cervical retrusion and capital flexion. So two things are going on at one time—flexion and extension. And although this is a relatively safe and developmental position, developmentally, it comes *after* we gain extension in the typical childhood developmental process.

“ *the average person sits 7.7 hours a day*

This overlooked fact is critically important in restoring control of our heads and our body's overall function.

Why?

Consider that the average person sits 7.7 hours a day. Some estimates have us close to 15 hours a day. And for many, that's in front of a computer. Sitting is essentially a return to the "womb state."

The body adapts to what it repeatedly does. So when you're always sitting (and looking down toward your computer) your body is stuck in flexion and the muscles that support your posture are no longer working to the degree they do when you are standing. This is especially true if you are sitting with a back support. Not only that, but your core musculature doesn't have to work either, so it becomes weak.

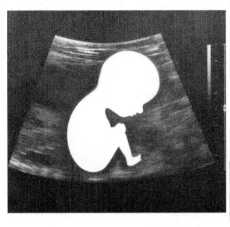 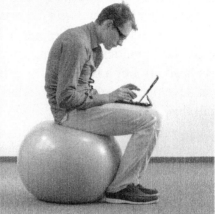

So when we stand, we end up standing with some weird lower back posture and a forward head posture, kind of like a chicken neck.

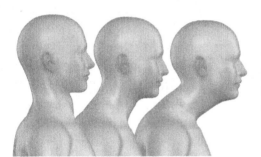

The further out the head is, the more it "weighs"—the more stress it places on the spine.

The path to restoration of posture—which coincidentally is a reflex—and the head control which determines it, is ***through extension, not flexion***. It may help to think of extension as looking up and flexion as looking down.

When you watch a child develop—not just watch one on a video or study pictures of one in books—but actually live with one 24/7, you'll notice one thing about a baby—he keeps his head up. His head position is determined by his eye position. Wherever his gaze is, his head follows. He looks up, his head follows, and his neck moves into extension. He looks down, and his neck moves into flexion. Look left or right? His head rotates. This is normal *and natural*. This strengthens his neck muscles, his upper and lower back, and his abs, especially in the early months when he's practicing "tummy time," lying on his stomach and keeping his head up. For a baby, learning how to control his head, is critical for his development of posture, balance, and coordination. Remember, we call this *strength*.

Again, this is a key concept to grasp: When you lose reflexive control of your head and neck, you'll notice poor posture, a loss of balance (one of the first signs of aging—*not deterioration due to a person's chronological age, but deterioration due to chronological neglect of movement*), and decreased coordination in everything from your reflexes to the visual tracking necessary to catch a ball to a loss of mobility in the rest of your joints, like the thoracic spine, shoulders, hips, and ankles.

We use head nods to begin regaining reflexive control of our heads. Head nods are very simple to perform. Our basic head nod starts on all fours—quadruped. (They can be performed in many other positions.) Simply look down and tuck your chin to your chest, keeping your arms straight then look up with your eyes and lift your head as high as you can, chin in the air. (Make sure to keep your tongue behind your teeth—its natural resting place—to protect your neck.) And repeat up and down and up and down and up and down.

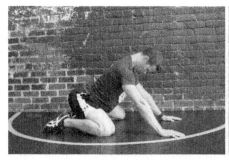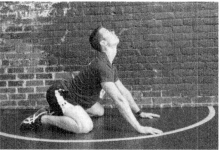

You'll find that head nods can unlock a sticky thoracic spine (an immobile upper back), grease or pry open rusty hips, and even help unlock frozen ankles. Such is the power of using your head!

Incidentally, posture improves and you no longer have to worry about using your cues. Posture, the posture you were designed to have when walking, just happens. Automatically. Like it's supposed to.

Somehow we've lost sight of this developmental process—the need and ability to control the head in any position and we have gone to what we call "artificial neutral"—or trying to keep the head and neck in its natural position during gait (walking) while performing other activities. We use terms like "neutral spine," and "long spine" and "pack the neck" to maintain the same head position we find while walking and transfer it into all other activities. This is not a good thing. We'll get into this concept in detail later. That's one of the points of neck nods: They help restore your reflexes so you don't have to worry about head and neck position. Your body does what comes naturally—what it's supposed to do without you having to think about it.

Why Do Head/Neck Nods Work?

Many fitness and healthcare professionals will see Head Nods and immediately condemn them because of what looks like the neck going into hyperextension (past normal joint end-range of motion). The truth is, that although we can use landmarks (creasing on the skin on the back of the neck) to give us some idea about what's going on inside the neck, we can't say for sure, without using something like a fluoroscope, which is machine that is like a moving x-ray.

This is an important observation to make because the neck it designed to extend—to move into extension. And by not doing moving it through it's full range of motion for fear of hyperextension, is a great way to handicap yourself.

And finally, the body is self-correcting: It's always trying to revert back to natural from normal. Normal is where you find yourself now, natural is where you're designed to live and function as an integrated system. So what may start as cervical hyperextension will quickly return to cervical extension as the vestibular system is activated and strengthened, and reflexive control is restored. And the more you do them, the faster this restoration process occurs.

> " *Head Nods not only restore posture, they can help your body's major systems (immune, digestive, cardiovascular, and respiratory systems) to not only function better, but to function optimally.*

Now that we have that out of the way, why exactly do Head/Neck Nods work? What is it that makes them such a powerful reset?

According to our "OS Science Guy," Dr. Mike Musselman, DC, a self-confessed "neuro-junkie," the Head Nods are incredibly powerful from a neuro-mechanical perspective because:

1. The specialized sensory cells of the upper cervical spine that communicate with your brain have a direct connection with the vestibular nuclei.
2. The vestibular nuclei are responsible for maintaining your upright posture.
3. Activation of these nuclei helps strengthen your postural patterns.
4. Due to the high number of these specialized sensory cells in the upper cervical spine, head movement is fantastic for brain nourishment.
5. Upper cervical spine sensory input has direct connections with the brain stem nuclei, which relays that information directly to the *nucleus tractus solitarious*, a part of the brain

that helps regulate the immune system, the gastrointestinal system, the heart, and the lungs.

6. Scientific evidence shows that input from the upper cervical spine is necessary for the proper regulation of these critically important body systems.

In layman's terms, Head Nods not only restore posture, they can help your body's major systems (immune, digestive, cardiovascular, and respiratory systems) to not only function better, but to function optimally.

Therefore, regaining head control by routinely performing Head/Neck Nods is critically important for your overall health and well-being.

Plus, they just feel durn good!

Keep Holding Your Tongue

Remember, the position of your tongue does matter. Placing your tongue in the "home" position, on the roof of your mouth behind your front teeth, is the reset within the RESETS.

In fact, placing the tongue on the roof of the mouth stimulates the tongue ligaments which are connected to the vestibular system.[27] It also frees up the neck's range of motion, engaging the hyoid muscle group on the front of the neck, which reduces shear forces in the cervical vertebrae. This is important, as moving the head and neck are what has the fastest, most direct impact on the vestibular system. If the vestibular system is activated and stimulated regularly, by moving the neck through its full range of motion, the whole body is improved; resulting in a sharper vestibular system, a more efficient brain, and a better moving, more connected, stronger body.

Did you know, people who rest their tongue on the bottom of their mouth tend to be mouth breathers AND, they also tend to have a forward head carriage? This means their head is not positioned above their shoulders as it should be. The more forward the head is held, the more the head "weighs" to the spine. If the head is tilted 15 degrees it places about 27 pounds of force on the spine. If the head is tilted 30 degrees, it places 40 pounds of force on the spine.[28] Remember, the adult head is only supposed to weigh about 10 pounds!

The placement of your little tongue can restore you. Keep your tongue where it belongs. This encourages diaphragmatic breathing, it helps restore your posture, and it allows your neck to move freely, as it should.

Keeping your tongue where it belongs is foundational to your overall health and wellbeing. This is why we call it the "reset within the reset."

Say "Yes" to Head Nods (get it?):

- Start on your hands and knees, like you're about to crawl (quadruped).
- Keep your mouth closed.
- Place (rest) your tongue on the roof of your mouth. (Again, if you're not sure exactly where this position is or how it should feel, just swallow, and your tongue will go there automatically.)
- Look down at the floor and tuck your chin to your chest.
- Look up at the ceiling and raise your head as high as your neck will allow you to move.
- Nod your head up and down. Lead with your eyes!
- DO NOT MOVE INTO PAIN OR DIZZINESS.
- Practice diaphragmatic breathing while performing your head nods—pausing and breathing in each position.
- Head Nods can be done while in the quadruped position on the forearms, the hands, while lying down, in a chair, or even while standing.

Keep Your Head Up

"While pregnant with my second child I had debilitating back, hip, and leg pain. This continued for over 3 years. The pain also traveled into my neck, causing numbness and issues in hands, feet, arms, legs and face. I also developed walking issues. One or both of my legs would give out (think drunk stumbling girl here) up to 100 times a day. My neck pain was so intense it was hard to lift my head off my pillow or look right and left.

I was sent to see 11 different doctors who told me I have/could have Multiple Sclerosis, Fibromyalgia, Ankylosing Spondylitis, Piriformis Syndrome, bulging discs and/or sciatica. I was also told exercising more would fix these issues. I was already lifting with kettlebells 3 times a week, walking, and participating in yoga or pilates on other days. I was confused, embarrassed, and hurting. After receiving treatment plans that contained only pain pills and muscle relaxers I was fed up.

Last February, I saw your video online speaking about relieving migraines by performing neck nods. I immediately tried them and have not looked back at the past once. I have looked up, down and sideways. I remedied myself with the daily five RESETS religiously and tried a chiropractor for the first time. I wanted a natural cure for this awful pain that had gone on for so long. I wanted to be off these medications. I wanted to play with my sweet babies without pain for the first time. Last June was my 9th and last chiropractic appointment as we were moving and I did not know of a chiropractor in our new town. I have not been back to a chiropractor since, but I continue to practice OS daily and I train with my kettlebells at least 3 times a week.

Last July, I received my MRI results showing all discs that had been bulging are totally normal and back in place! The pain became less and less, and now coming up on a year later, I am totally pain free! I had forgotten what it was like not to hurt! It does not hurt to sit, stand, drive or hold my children! My walking has also improved. My legs have only given out 7 times in the last four months. I am off all pain medications and muscle relaxers. In short, I have experienced a miracle!

I know God does not make mistakes and He led me to OS for a reason. I want to tell the world what I have experienced! If I can help one person learn how to ease pain through all of this it will have been worth the years of hurting.

I wish doctors knew how to recommend such a movement system, especially for mommies. I tell everyone I know and they all want to learn about OS. Every time I show someone the RESETS they laugh. I believe it is the God given movement patterns and childlike quality that causes this. As laughter is the best medicine, I will continue to show everyone OS and will practice it for life.

Thank you for giving me this gift and please let me know how to bring it to others. Thank you for taking the time to read my story and may God Bless you!"

Sincerely,
Amber Harrison, mom
Georgia

"P.S. I'm sorry if this is too wordy and long, I tried to condense it. THREE years is a long time and I was told so many different things by doctors I wasn't sure what all to put in here. Thank you again for listening and for your time :)"

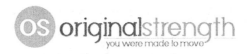

Know Your Roll

Before Tim's first son, Luke, could crawl, Tim would often place him on the floor in the middle of the room, thinking he was safe from objects that might harm him. Tim would then get distracted by chores or hobbies that desired his attention. Tim did this until Luke discovered how to roll. Once Luke learned how to silently roll anywhere he wanted to go in the room, Tim's days of getting distracted by his chores and hobbies were over. Luke demanded his full attention. He was like a rolling ninja.

One time, while Tim was working on his computer, he turned around to a huge surprise. He was expecting to find Luke behind him, where he placed him, but Luke wasn't there. He had rolled to the other side of the room. It was an impressive distance. Apparently something over there had caught his attention. Luke, like most babies, learned how to roll to get to places he wanted to go.

Rolling is how we learn to get to the objects that beg for our curiosity. It is the true foundation of our gait pattern, as it is our first method of locomotion. When a child learns how to roll, he begins further tying his X together. Building on top of the strength that breathing and learning head control develop, rolling is where the child starts connecting the opposite shoulder to the opposite hip, anteriorly and posteriorly (rolling connects the front side of your X and the back side of your X). It adds another layer of strength to the child's center.

When a child rolls, he is developing rotational strength and stability. This is the strength that prepares his body for the rotational forces walking and running produce. This rotational stability also allows the child's trunk to remain stable under asymmetrical and contralateral loads. This is a critical component of spine health. This rotational strength is also the reflexive strength that allows him to balance and command control over his movements.

Remembering how to roll around on the floor is a key to returning the strength we were designed to have. Everything it does for the developing child, still holds true for the "redeveloping" adult. It is also worth mentioning here that rolling is crucial to keeping your spine young and healthy. In case you have forgotten, your spine was made to rotate!

> " *rolling is crucial to keeping your spine young and healthy*

Adults should be able to easily roll around on the floor just like children can. However, this is not always the case, as we have often witnessed during the Original Strength Screen and Assessment (OSSA). In the OSSA, rolling can quickly reveal how well connected a person's body really is; whether or not their shoulders are connected to their hips, and whether or not they have their rotational strength and stability, among other things. Again, we should all be able to roll around on the floor with ease. But don't be fooled by the "ease". Effortless rolling is a sign of tremendous strength and health! A fluid X is a strong X.

Love Your Brain

Rolling doesn't just tie the X together. It builds significantly more than reflexive strength. It also builds a very healthy brain. When you roll, you are greatly activating your vestibular system. You are also stimulating your skin, the largest sensory organ you posses. Your skin receives all kinds of information about you and your environment: Such as how cold you are, hot humid it is, what kind of surface you are touching, how hard something is touching you, etc.. Some even refer to the skin as the "outer brain" because it receives so much information. In fact, the skin contains 640,000 sensory receptors connected to the spinal cord by over 500,000 neural pathways![29] It is like a great big nerve in and of itself.

Your brain craves information about you and your surroundings. Not receiving this information is the same as starving your brain. In fact, scientists have learned children that don't receive loving touch from a care giver actually suffer from the same effects as undernourishment including retarded bone growth, poor muscular coordination, immunological weakness, and general apathy.[30] In case you are wondering, a "loving touch" can be someone rocking a child to sleep, calming a child by rubbing their back, or simply playing with a child. It provides tactile information to the brain as well as positional information about the child's body.

" *the skin is like a great big nerve in and of itself.*

Rolling, much like loving touch, provides the brain with this same, nourishing information. Remember, your vestibular system receives all sensory information from the body and sends this information to the brain. All the stimulation and activation that rolling generates, literally feeds your brain with nourishment. Every time you roll, you give your brain rich information that either creates new neural connections (nerve pathways in your brain) or cements the neural connections you already have. The more neural connections you have, and the more cemented they are, the more efficient your brain becomes, allowing for quicker thought, and quicker processing of incoming information. This keeps your brain healthy, allowing you to become a better thinker and a better mover.

Rolling doesn't just help make you stronger, it helps to make you whole. But then, so does loving touch.

How Do You Roll?

Rolling is simply the act of lying on the floor and transitioning from your belly to your back and from your back to your belly. There are more ways to roll than there are letters in the alphabet. But first, because it works wonders in restoring reflexive strength and movement patterns, we will look at rolling the way Gray Cook outlines in his book, *Movement*.

Segmental Rolling:[31]

- Back to Belly Rolling—Upper Body:
  - Lie on your back with your legs straight and your arms straight over head.
  - **Using your head,** neck and right arm, reach across your body as far as you can and roll to your belly. **Do not cheat and use your legs!**
  - Can you do this with equal movement and effort with both arms?

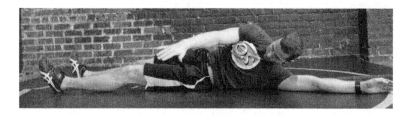

- Belly to Back Rolling—Upper Body:
    - Lie on your belly with your legs straight and your arms straight overhead.
    - **Use your head**, neck and right arm to reach back across your body and roll to your back. **Do not cheat and use your legs!**
    - Can you do this with equal movement and effort with both arms?

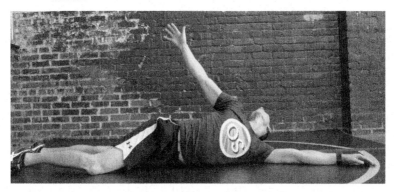

- Back to Belly Rolling—Lower Body:
    - Lie on your back with your legs straight and your arms straight over head.
    - Using your right leg, reach across your body and roll to your belly. **Do not cheat and use your arms!**
    - Can you do this with equal movement and effort with both legs?

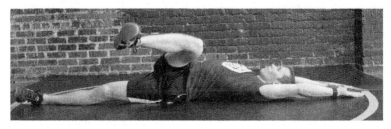

- Belly to Back Rolling—Lower Body:
  - Lie on your belly with your legs straight and your arms straight over head.
  - Use your right leg to reach back across your body and roll to your back. **Do not cheat and use your arms!**
  - Can you do this with equal movement and effort with both legs?

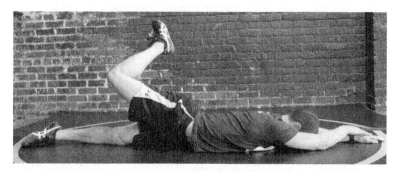

Even though babies don't roll as deliberate as Tim is doing in the pictures, they do segmentally roll. They are extremely fluid and they roll piece by piece, almost like an ocean wave. You should be able to roll this way too.

The segmental roll is a great place to start when it comes to rolling. We like to start with this method because it can both expose movement issues and unlock movement issues at the same time. At the Original Strength Institute, we have witnessed rolling "fix", or cleanup an entire Functional Movement Screen Score[32] in several of our clients. This makes sense because rolling is programmed deep inside our original operating system. It is one of the first ways we start to learn and develop our movements and movement patterns as infants. It can also be a great way to relearn and rebuild them again as adults.

There are eight rolling patterns involved in the segmental roll: belly to back, back to belly, left to right, right to left, right arm, left arm, right leg, and left leg. Ideally, all eight of those patterns should be of equal ease. In truth, they should all be fluid and effortless. However, in some people, some of these patterns may be difficult. In other people, some of these patterns may not even be currently possible at all—they can't roll.

Often times, simply spending time on the floor, exploring the segmental roll, can restore these patterns. Rolling makes *rolling* better. In other times, the segmental roll may need to be broken down into smaller bits and pieces we call regressions. These regressions are explored in detail at the *Original Strength* workshops.

Once segmental rolling can be performed with ease, other forms of rolling can be introduced. The following rolls are more advanced rolls. These are just examples of different ways to roll. They need not be performed if pressing the RESET button on the body is all that is desired. However, they may make the RESET button even stronger. These rolling variations also provide a fun, playful way to explore the body's movement capabilities while at the same time, they sharpen and improve the body's ability to move.

The Head Roll:

- While resting on your forearms and belly, use only your head and neck and roll over to your back with your legs straight and your arms resting over your chest.

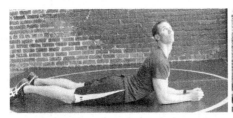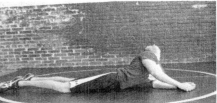

- While lying on your back, use only your head and neck and roll to your belly.
  - You can "land" propped up on your forearms.

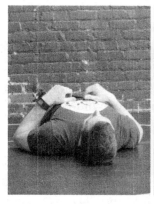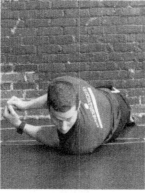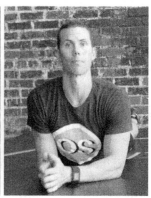

- Practice rolling in both directions.
- This is an upper body segmental roll without the use of the arms.

This is just one way to perform a head roll. Babies actually employ a different type of head roll that we LOVE to do. However, because of the nature in which that particular head roll is performed, we only demonstrate and teach it in public at our workshops.

The Elevated Roll:

- Assume the push-up position on your hands and feet.
- Use your right leg to reach back across your body and roll until your right foot rests on the ground.
- As you reach and roll with your right leg, your right hand will leave the ground.
- When your right foot makes contact with the ground, your right arm should end up pointing up at the sky.
- Push both feet into the ground and reach for the sky with your pelvis.
- When you are ready to return, REACH across your body with your right arm and drive it down towards the ground. This will pull your lower body back over to the starting push-up position.

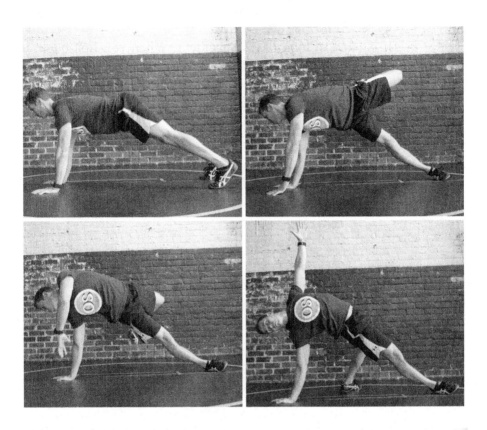

The elevated roll feels fantastic! It can make a great "movement snack" to throw into your day every now and then.

Rolling Tips

- Remember the body is designed to follow the head, and the head is designed to follow the eyes! When rolling from the upper body, lead with your eyes and use your head.
- Keep your mouth closed.
- Place (rest) your tongue on the roof of your mouth.
- To roll fluidly and segmentally, you have to be able to "let go" and relax your body. If you haven't mastered diaphragmatic breathing yet, this may be next to impossible.
- DO NOT MOVE INTO PAIN. You can roll to the edge of it,

but don't roll into it.
- It is okay to look like an accident. When you first begin to roll, it may not look so fluid. This is okay. Keep rolling. With time and effort, fluidity will come.

The Impact of Rolling

"I've said it, and I'll say it again, I found rolling long ago, actually studying psychology and neurology. I was lucky enough to realize the physical and 'life impact' value, and through digging, and stumbling onto Original Strength very early on. There is still nothing I have found that has had as big of an impacting on correcting my clients movement, living life, and just flat out being bad asses."

–Matt Woodard, A.K.A. Kal-El
Florida

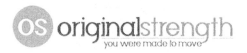

Rocking Yourself Together

Have you ever watched a child learn how to crawl? After they have built a good amount of strength from spending time on the floor, lifting their heads and rolling around, they begin to try to push up from the ground to get up on their hands and knees. Once they get to their hands and knees, they want to go. But they can't. Often, when a child builds the strength to get to their hands and knees, they have to start building the strength to maintain that position, and they have to start building coordination.

It takes a great deal of coordination to get all four limbs to cooperate in order to crawl. Even if a child is not a crawler, but a "scooter," it still takes strength and coordination for them to master their preferred method of getting from one place to another.

Rocking back and forth is how a child builds this strength and coordination. It is pretty cool to witness a child doing this. It almost looks as if they are trying to build enough momentum to get their body to crawl; like they are trying to overcome the inertia of being motionless.

What a child is really doing when they rock back and forth is assembling their entire body as one whole unit. Rocking is the primitive pattern that really starts to integrate the entire body. It teaches the brain the body is one whole piece and not several bits and pieces. When a person rocks, child or adult, all the major joints start moving together as one unit. The joints of the feet, the ankles, the knees, the hips, the spine, the shoulders, the wrist—they all move together in unison and they become integrated into the brain.

But this is just what joints do. Rocking also further reflexively integrates the muscles of the body. When a child rocks back and forth on his hands and knees, he is reflexively building stability throughout his body. His rotator cuffs learn how to stabilize the shoulder joints, he builds stability in his scapula and pelvis, his postural muscles learn how to stabilize the spine, and his prime movers learn how to coordinate movement between his limbs. Rocking teaches the shoulders and hips how to work together.

" posture is a reflexive position you have, not a position you try to hold with muscular effort

Rocking is also the motion, and position, that *reflexively* sets a person's posture. Remember, posture is a reflexive position you have, not a position you try to hold with muscular effort. It should just *be*. The quadruped position, being on the hands and knees, is where the cervical curve (the neck curve) and the lumbar curve (the lower back curve) get set. This is the position that sets the shape of our spine and teaches our core muscles how to reflexively respond in order to maintain optimal posture. In fact, we actually use rocking inside of the Original Strength Screen and Assessment (OSSA) to quickly determine the state of a person's postural reflexes.

Rocking is a powerful reset. It assembles and integrates the entire body and soul as one.

Rocking Soothes the Soul

Rocking does not just integrate the body, it also integrates the soul with the body. Your soul—your mind, your thoughts and your emotions—is also greatly effected by how your body moves. A mind that doesn't receive movement can become a restless, agitated, mind. You already know this to be true.

> " *Your soul—your mind, your thoughts and your emotions— is also greatly effected by how your body moves.*

What does every mother intuitively know how to do to soothe an upset child? What do agitated children do that are having trouble with their emotions? What does an irate adult do who is perhaps ready to fight? They rock, or sway, or pace. It is all the same, they move back and forth to soothe and calm their emotions. Rocking back and forth is a program buried deep inside of you. It stimulates your vestibular system, it nourishes your brain, and it can calm the storms within you. It can "RESET" your emotions.

As we learned earlier, the brain craves input. Stimulating the vestibular system nourishes the brain and body as much as good food nourishes the brain and body. It is movement that keeps the nerves from "unraveling". Is it any wonder that so many Americans are so frazzled and stressed out? We live in a world that encourages not moving. If a movement like rocking back and forth can help reduce and relieve stress, then the opposite is also true. Not moving, being still most of the day, can perpetuate stress and exasperate the mind. How easy is it to think and make rational decisions when you are upset? Press RESET. Rock yourself to peace.

By the way, mothers also hum or sing soft lullabies to their crying children as they rock them. Humming greatly stimulates the vestibular system.[33] Mom is not only calming her upset child. She is also doing two things that help to soothe her nerves as well.

The next time you get upset, try humming while you rock. You may find that it works wonders to settle you.

Rock On

Rocking seems to be the high payoff reset for most people. We have seen it restore ankle mobility, hip mobility, relieve lower back pain and discomfort, and correct many other movement issues. Even our good friend and famous author, Dan John, credits rocking to regaining his strength and rehabbing his hip after having undergone hip surgery. Today Dan is competing in the Highland Games and he is enjoying Olympic Lifting, his passion. Rocking helped Dan rebuild his body and regain his *original strength!* Dan even told me rocking seemed to calm and relax him. If you knew Dan, you would know he is full throttle, high energy and passionate. If he says rocking calms him, that is a powerful testimony!

Rocking is performed by getting down on your hands and knees, keeping a BIG chest, with the crown of your head pointed towards the sky (hold your head up). From this position, simply push your butt back towards your feet. Then, rock forward placing your weight back over your hands. Back and forth, back and forth…

In the beginning, try it nice and slow. As you get comfortable with it, you can play with the speed in which you rock. As your hips loosen up, you can also play with the width in which you place your knees by moving them closer together or farther apart. You can also rock using different foot positions. There really is not "one way" to rock. Playing with the different rocking positions can be very relaxing and therapeutic.

Be sure to hold your head up when rocking. When a child rocks back and forth, his head is held up. Yours should be, too. Remember that the body is designed to follow the head; you are reflexively wired together by the movements of your head. In fact, you can see for yourself how this works. From the bottom rocking position, perform some neck nods while you are sitting back towards your calves. You will feel your whole back musculature "turn on." If you try to look over your shoulders to see your own butt, you will even feel your lats (big "muscle wings" on your back) and the muscles around your scapula pull your shoulder blades down towards your butt. Head position initiates the reflexive actions of your postural muscles.

Rocking back and forth also engages the pelvic floor; it causes the pelvic floor muscles to fire reflexively. You may notice this as you push your butt back towards your calves. Especially if you increase the speed in which your rock. A reflexively strong pelvic floor is essential for overall strength and health.

Original strength starts from the inside out. It happens between a properly functioning diaphragm and a properly functioning pelvic floor. Remember, the diaphragm and the pelvic floor form the inner core, they make the center of you, the X, solid. If the diaphragm is working well because we are breathing properly, and the pelvic floor is functioning well reflexively, then the X is very strong. Performing diaphragmatic breathing along with rocking can be a very powerful reset, especially for women trying to restore their bodies after child birth. Men, it is a powerful reset for you, too! Again, a properly functioning, reflexively strong pelvic floor is essential for obtaining optimal strength. Believe it or not, your body was designed to express optimal strength.

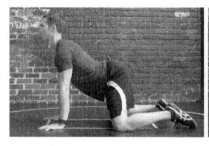 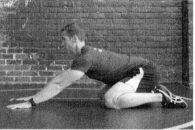

How to Perform Rocking:

- Start on your hands and knees as if you are about to crawl.
- In the beginning, place the tops of your feet on the ground (plantarflex your feet—laces down!)
- Keep a "big" chest, like Billy Bodybuilder on the beach.
- Hold your head up so that you can see the horizon.
- Push your butt back towards your feet. (Bottom Position)
  - Play with head nods while holding the bottom position of the rock.
  - Play with diaphragmatic breathing while holding the bottom position of the rock.
- Move in and out, back and forth, slowly—at first.
  - Play with different speeds as you get used to the motion.
  - Play with different width positions for your knees.

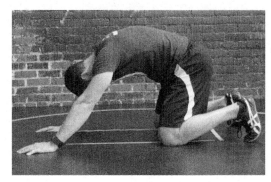

This is not what we want to do. Notice that the head is down and the spine is round. Keep the head up and keep the spine "flat" by holding a proud chest.

If you have the strength, and you want to add a little extra resistance to rocking, you can perform elevated rocking, on your hands and your feet. This places a much greater demand on your muscles as it greatly increases the tension placed on them (your full bodyweight). It's all reflexive. You don't have to think about tightening your muscles, it happens automatically. This is an "easy" way to build strength and integrate your whole body. It's a *strong* RESET...

Rocking on Hands and Feet

- Start on your hands and feet.
- Keep a tall chest, like Billy Bodybuilder on the beach.
- Hold your head up so you can see the horizon.
- Push your butt back towards your feet.
    - Make sure you keep a BIG chest!!!
    - Make sure you breathe! Do not hold your breath.
- Move in and out, back and forth, slowly—at first.
    - Play with different speeds as you get used to the motion.

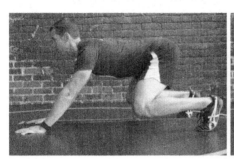 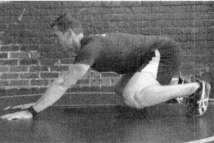

Movement is More Than a Physical Exercise

"I've completed my first month of "Bulletproof Training" (OS was first called Becoming Bulletproof). Of twenty-four scheduled training days, I've trained twenty. I have done RESETS daily and sometimes several times daily.

I start each day upon awaking giving grace, then performing RESETS as I set on the edge of my bed. Breathing, head nods, rocking, and cross crawls. This is the best I have felt all year and the best I have felt spiritually, physically and emotionally in a very long time.

I'm looking forward to my continued progress and journey of becoming the best person I can be and enjoying life to its fullest. I want to thank you for your help and guidance in my journey.

Be Blessed, Be Strong, Be Happy"

–Kirby Sams
Austin TX

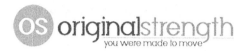

The Whole Foundation

After a child relentlessly builds his strength through the consistent effort of pushing himself up, away from the floor, he is ready to begin crawling. Crawling is the moving culmination of all the other developmental movements we've covered. It is diaphragmatic breathing, combined with head control, combined with rotary stability, combined with the integration of rocking. It is the developmental movement that establishes THE foundation of the most graceful and capable creature to ever grace the planet—You.

> " *It is the developmental movement
> that establishes THE foundation of the
> most graceful and capable creature
> to ever grace the planet—You.*

Crawling ties *everything* together; through motion. And when we say "everything" we mean everything!

Pressing Reset With Cross-Lateral Movements

Crawling is a cross-lateral movement and it completes the foundation of the human gait pattern. (Remember, rolling is where we begin locomotion.) When we crawl or walk, our opposite limbs are supposed to move in coordination with each other. This is the design of the X. It is this coordinated movement that ties the brain together, it ties the body together, and ties the brain and body together.

How does crawling tie the brain together?

Crawling combines two halves to make a whole. Your brain has two hemispheres, the right hemisphere, known as the gestalt side, and the left hemisphere, known as the logic side. For your body to be efficient at anything, both hemispheres need to work well together.[34] Performing cross-lateral movements and/or midline crossing movements increases the communication between the two hemispheres of your brain.[35] Midline crossing movements are movements that cross the middle line of your body. For example, taking your right hand and reaching for your left leg is a midline crossing movement.

Cross-lateral and midline crossing movements can actually cause the brain to make new neural connections between the two hemispheres. They literally tie the brain together by creating new neural connections inside the brain. This is what makes cross-lateral and midline crossing movements crucial for learning and brain development. These movements are also crucial for physical development. The more neural connections there are between the two hemispheres, the better the hemispheres work together and communicate with the body. This results in the ability for the body to express its full movement and strength potential.

Crawling is not a new fad or fitness craze. Nor is it a recent evolutionary development in humans. It is part of the original gait template programmed into your great, great, great grandfather. Since man was, crawling has been pre-programmed inside of man's operating system.

It refreshes the nervous system and it restores and optimizes our whole design.

We were all programmed to crawl. However, not all of us do. For various reasons like germaphobic parents who were afraid to put their child on the floor, or over enthusiastic parents who rushed their kids into walking, or cultural norms, or simply having no space to crawl, some children skip crawling, or don't spend enough time crawling. Research has shown that those who skip crawling are more likely to have learning disorders.[36] They are more likely to have movement and coordination issues as well because crawling sets the foundation for the gait pattern. Research has also shown that crawling can help a person overcome learning disorders, if not be healed from them.

Maybe you were a person who didn't crawl. It doesn't matter. The program is still inside of you and you can still "run the program" and reset your nervous system, rebuild your brain, and restore your *original strength*. Even if you are 99 years young and you haven't really used that program for the last 88 years, it is still inside of you.

Crawling sharpens your neural pathways and their ability to send and receive signals, making your reflexes not only more efficient but much faster. This is how crawling physically ties the X together, building and restoring effortless strength and mobility. For example, through mechanoreceptors, nerve endings, in the hands and feet, crawling stimulates reflexive core musculature activation, which gets the shoulders and pelvis working together.[37] In *The Well Balanced Child*, Sally Goddard Blythe points out that "Movement on all fours (like rocking and crawling) also helps to align the spine at the back of the neck with the sacral region in preparation for proper alignment in the upright posture."[38] Every single step that is made when crawling stimulates these mechanoreceptors, thus stimulating the reflexive core muscular activation that connects the torso, aligns the spine and establishes optimal upright posture. In truth, crawling reflexively stimulates all the muscles throughout your body. Just watch a person's triceps contract when they crawl. Every step they take with their hands elicits a contraction in their triceps, AND all the other muscles in their body you can't even see. Can you see the gentle strength training taking place here?

Crawling is what enables us to express our full athleticism, even in ways you wouldn't necessarily think about. It can improve your binocular vision, your hand-eye coordination, and even your binaural hearing (your perception of sound from two ears).[39] Crawling helps lay the foundation, on multiple levels, of who we become and how we express ourselves through movement. Crawling is the movement program that enables us to become capable—of anything.

Geoff didn't crawl (much) as a child and always had trouble catching and throwing, and therefore opted for more "hands on" sports such as wrestling and weightlifting. One of his "in-home," long-time clients, a former baseball catcher, used to love to "torture" Geoff by throwing balls at him, only to watch Geoff fumble all over himself to catch, and more often than not, ultimately drop the ball. One day, his client threw a ball at him, only this time Geoff didn't even look to catch the ball. He simply spotted the ball with his peripheral vision, reached out, and plucked it out of the air with his left hand. This arrested his client's attention. And it opened the door for his client to start using and benefiting from *Original Strength*, eliminating his chronic lower back issues.

With all this attention we are giving to crawling, this may be a thought that keeps running through your head: *But babies learn to crawl so they can walk. We were designed to walk on two feet. Babies progress to walking! We are not supposed to keep crawling around as adults!*

This is true. But it is also true that **we are not supposed to sit around all day, either.**

And yet, that is what most of us do.

Yes, walking and running are both cross-lateral movements requiring coordination and they should incorporate both hemispheres of our brains. But, you know what?

You can fake walking and running. People do it all the time. They walk and run without using their shoulders and arms properly. Some people walk around without even using their arms at all. They aren't moving according to their design. As a result, they don't have the solid foundation they were made to have and they cannot express their bodies full strength and mobility potential. They are limited, and therefore, they are not as resilient and capable as they should be.

> " *You can fake walking and running...*
>
> *...But, a person cannot fake crawling.*

But, a person cannot fake crawling. It is deliberate. Their shoulders and hips have to work together in order to get from one place to another. Crawling RESETS the nervous system and returns walking to the cross-lateral gait pattern it was meant to be. When a person walks as they were designed, walking becomes a reset; THE reset we were all made to do, all the time.

Learning to Crawl

When it comes to crawling, use patience and GOOD judgment. Just because you think one type of crawl may look "cooler," or "sexier" than another, you need to spend time crawling *where you are; at the level your body is currently able.* We have to say this because many people want to jump right into the Spider-man crawl, but their bodies may not be ready for the demands of the Spider-man crawl. Believe it or not, some people are not ready for the demands of baby crawling, either.

> " *you need to start where you are, at the level your body is ready to handle.*

The point is, you need to start where you are, at the level your body is ready to handle. The Spider-man crawl is awesome and it can build the strength of your dreams, but so can the baby crawl—if you'll explore it with patience, honesty and curiosity.

If you are in doubt as to which crawl to start with, simply start with the baby crawl (hands and knees) and own it before you move on to the hand and foot crawls we are about to share with you. If you cannot meet or maintain the guidelines for baby crawling, try starting with the commando crawl (on your forearms and thighs). Start where your body will let you begin…

Commando Crawling

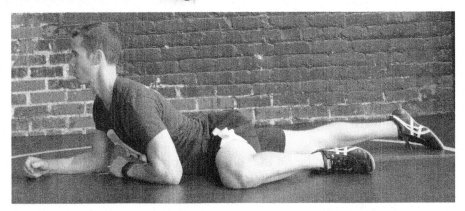

- Lie on your belly and prop yourself up on your forearms.
- Stay "tall"—do not let your neck sink or sag between your shoulder blades.
- Hold your head up.
- Drag your opposite leg in coordination with your opposite arm.

Baby Crawling

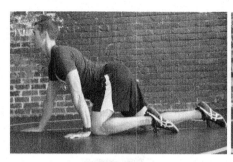 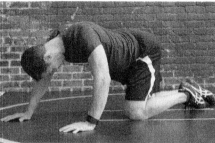

Like this   Not like this

- Get on your hands and knees.
- Hold your head up so you can see where you are going.
- Keep a "big" chest.
- Move your opposite limbs in coordination with each other.
    - The knees should track underneath your body, inside your arms.
- Drag your feet.
- Keep your tongue on the roof of your mouth!
- Try to maintain breathing through your nose.

Leopard Crawling

After baby crawling, we introduce leopard crawling. Leopard crawling looks very similar to baby crawling except leopard crawling is on the hands and feet. The head, spine and butt look just as they did in the baby crawl. Leopard crawling should look fluid and strong, *like* a leopard.

The leopard crawl is a progression to the baby crawl and a regression to the Spider-man crawl. In the leopard crawl, the knees track underneath the body and inside the arms, just as they do in the baby crawl. This is a great way to crawl in order to build reflexive strength in your center (your X) and ensure your body is ready for the Spider-man crawl.

The Spider-man crawl takes a very high degree of core muscle coordination developed only through high levels of reflexive stability, something most people who sit all day don't have. For those who attempt to Spider-man crawl before they should, it is evident that their bodies are not yet ready. Their hips move all wobbly, flopping from side to side, and most of their movement comes from rotating at their lumbar spine. This is not good. Especially if they have ever had a lower back injury or lower back pain. Because of his own hip and lower back injuries, Geoff literally spent two years performing the Leopard crawl before he could successfully transition to the Spider-man crawl.

Remember, be patient, be honest with yourself, and use good judgment.

By the way, just because we say leopard crawling is a regression to Spider-man crawling does not mean it is easier. Leopard crawling is much more demanding from a mental and physical standpoint. It requires more steps to go the same distance as Spider-man crawling. Your legs, hips, core, heart and lungs will not enjoy it nearly as much as they do Spider-man crawling.

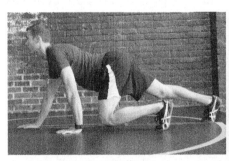 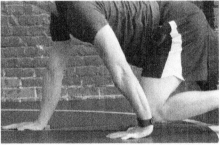

- Get on your hands and feet.
- Hold your head up so you can see where you are going.
- Keep a "big" chest.
- Keep your butt down, below your head.
  - Do not let your butt rise up above your head.
- Move your opposite limbs in coordination with each other.
  - The knees should track underneath your body, inside your

arms.

- Stay long and take small steps with your legs until you are strong enough to maintain a flat back and take the longer steps that would actually put your knees inside your arms.
- Keep your tongue on the roof of your mouth!
- Try to maintain breathing through your nose.

Spider-man Crawling

"*Holding the butt down low and keeping the head up demands strength from the body's center.*

As mentioned above, Spider-man crawling is a progression from leopard crawling. In the Spider-man crawl, the knees now track outside the elbows. The head, spine, and butt should remain in the same relationship they did in both the baby crawl and leopard crawl. However, the Spider-man crawl takes the hips through a much greater range of motion and it requires a great deal more reflexive strength and stability to keep the pelvis level with the ground; it really challenges your rotational stability.

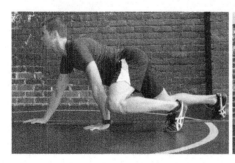 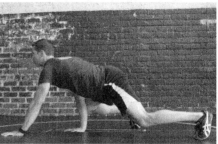

When the body is able to effortlessly handle the demands of this rotational challenge, the body is strong, powerful and capable.

- Get on your hands and feet.
- Hold your head up so you can see where you are going.
- Keep a "big" chest.
- Keep your butt down, below your head.
  - Do not let your butt rise up above your head.
- Move your opposite limbs in coordination with each other.
  - The knees should track outside your arms.
- Keep your tongue on the roof of your mouth!
- Try to maintain breathing through your nose.

Crawling for Superhuman Strength

Believe it or not, crawling can give you superhuman strength; especially, crawling on your hands and your feet. Both leopard and Spider-man crawling are tremendous strength builders. They are probably the best way to really tie the body together—from a strength standpoint as well as a neurological standpoint. You can actually RESET your body and build a super-strong body at the same time.

One of the reasons these two crawls are so beneficial is they both keep the butt held down, below the head, and the head is held up. Just holding your body in this position takes strength. Getting used to being in this position builds strength. Every time your hands and feet—especially if you are barefoot—touch the ground, you reinforce reflexive strength and dynamic stability by putting pressure on the proprioceptors (nerves) in your palms and feet.

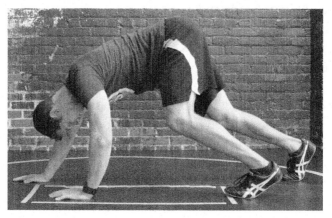

This is not what we want to do. Keep that butt down!

Notice, again, the butt is held down low. This is not what we call a bear crawl. In a bear crawl, the butt pops up and the head drops down. When this happens, the center of the X is no longer under tension, and the restorative, reflexive postural benefits are lost. Holding the butt down low and keeping the head up demands strength from the body's center. In fact, when people tire from leopard or Spider-man crawling, their butts will pop up, like a turkey thermometer. If the butt pops up, the abs are done and the turkey is cooked! Bear crawls can be good, but they are not "best." Keep your butt down and build your strength.

How can you build a super strong body with crawling?

Simple. You spend time crawling. You can actually crawl as your entire strength training session. Be warned, this may not be as easy as you think it will be. Try leopard or Spider-man crawling for 5 straight minutes. If you can achieve one minute off the bat, that's impressive! If you try this, you will quickly notice that crawling takes strength, stamina, a good heart and a great set of lungs. The good news is crawling like this builds all of these things, *especially if you hold your tongue on the roof of your mouth and breathe in and out of your nose.* This is not easy to do, but it can become easy over time.

We often ask people, "If you could leopard crawl for 10 straight minutes, without stopping, what can you not do?" The answer is, "You can do anything you want to do." Why? Because you are as strong as you could ever want to be. You have real strength. You have the ability to tackle and overcome physical obstacles. Strength, stamina, will power, focus, tenacity, ability; crawling for 10 minutes develops and delivers all of these qualities. Please understand, we are not recommending you crawl for 10 minutes. We are only eluding to the possibility that you are capable of doing so.

Your body already has everything inside of it that you could ever need to become powerful, strong and resilient. You are never limited. You can progress your crawling by increasing time and distance. Or you can change directions (forward, backward, sideways, in circles…) and change speeds. You can even add resistance. You don't need a room full of weights, machines, and gadgets. You can crawl. You can do it anywhere. It is low skill. It is not dangerous. Heck, if you fall, you're already on the ground! The point is, you were made to crawl, and crawling was intended to make you strong.

If you want to express your full strength potential, find a place for crawling in your life. Leopard and/or Spider-man crawling build ridiculous strength. But then, so does baby crawling. Do not miss the simplicity of these beautiful movements. It doesn't really matter how you crawl, just crawl—often. Yes, people will stare. It does not matter. Superhuman strength is not afraid. It is courageous. It stands out and people take notice.

I Climbed a Mountain

"I climbed a mountain this year. Something I didn't think I would be able to do again and I owe it in large part to Original Strength and one of their trainers Trevor Trebbien.

I have been a massage therapist for about 22 years. Have learned and taught about movement and how to take care of one's self for many years. Due to my own history and background I've always loved taking care of others; it was always easier than taking care of myself.

By the time I realized all the activities I wasn't doing any more like hiking, dancing, or even walking much, my body decided it was time to make me pay attention. 2 years ago my right hip literally gave out on me. Long story short, it changed everything. After a visit to the ER and learning I had severe arthritis to the point of holes in my bones and nothing left for cushion in the joints, both hips got replaced within 6 weeks of each other. One surgery went really well and one did not. I couldn't walk, work, or even go back to my own home due to not being able to navigate stairs, and I wasn't even 50 yet.

As great as my Physical therapists were, they had gone as far as they could and I still needed something more. Discovering a Cross Fit groupon coupon, I decided to try Trevor's gym and once again everything in my life was about to change; this time for the better.

When I learned about The Original Strength program and the key part about learning to crawl, I had no idea of the far reaching implications it would have. The spark created by re-patterning my body and brain to move forward in a healthy way started to seep into every part of my being and how I chose to live.

Through the Original Strength work and the help of Trevor and his staff, I gained a life that I had almost forgotten about. I learned that I could be strong again.

Re-patterning and learning to crawl has became a mantra for my mental, emotional, and spiritual being as well. It was a key for me that unlocked my life. I realized I could go from crawling to moving forward to climbing mountains.

It doesn't get better than that as far as I'm concerned and I am so grateful."

–Corrine Ranard
Portland Oregon

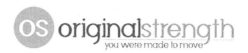

Crossing the Line

As powerful as crawling can be, it is not the most powerful reset. That designation is reserved for cross-crawls. Cross-crawls are done by simply touching opposite limbs together. To do this, you have to cross the midline of your body. This is a very deliberate action, like crawling. You can't fake this!

Cross-crawls are nothing new. They have been around for years. You probably even did them when you were a child in P.E. class or when you participated in warm-ups at your team practices. For most of us, this was the extent of our cross-crawl performance. They were simply a movement we used very briefly to prepare for other physical activities. We did them, but we didn't know their benefits. Well, some people knew. Chiropractors like Dr. Leroy Perry, the first chiropractor ever to serve as an Olympic Team Doctor, have always known they benefit the body. Yet, as far as physical health goes, cross-crawls have pretty much remained unnoticed throughout the years.

In the world of brain development and rehabilitation, cross-crawls have long been used to treat learning disabilities in children as well as help stroke patients regain their normal function. Can you imagine? Touching the right hand to the left leg and touching the left hand to the right leg is powerful enough to create new neural connections in a damaged brain and restore function to a person's body.

Remember, crossing the midline of the body, performing cross-crawls, has many of the same brain benefits crawling does. Here is a secret: if cross-crawls share many of the same brain benefits as crawling, they share many of the same physical benefits as well.

Why are cross-crawls the most powerful reset?

Because anyone, regardless of their physical condition, can perform some type of cross-crawl. Not everyone can get down on the floor and crawl like a baby. Not everyone will be able to remember how to use their diaphragm when they breathe. But anyone and everyone can perform a cross-crawl. And when they do, miracles can happen.

We have seen people who haven't been able to stand on their own, out of their own chairs and able to stand up, unassisted, after learning how to perform cross-crawls.

> *anyone, regardless of their physical condition, can perform some type of cross-crawl.*

We've even seen people go from needing a walker to walking on their own after learning how to do cross-crawls.

Cross-crawls are the simplest, most powerful, most accessible and most restorative reset there is. It is the most accessible reset because anyone can do it. It is the most restorative reset because of the hope it can give a person. Hope is powerful. It restores strength and courage.

Focusing With Your Tongue

One nice benefit of performing cross-crawls is that they increase focus and mental alertness. They can make a nice movement snack that helps remove mental fogginess and they can help fight away the sleep monster. If you can't find a cup of coffee, you can always make a quick cross-crawl.

Like cross-crawls, the position of your tongue can also increase mental alertness. Because the tongue stimulates the vestibular system, it also activates the RAS (the Reticular Activating System) which increases focus and balance.[40] The RAS is responsible for regulating arousal and sleep-wake transitions in people. Holding the tongue on the roof of your mouth, and even pressing the tongue against the roof of your mouth, can stimulate the RAS system and make you more alert, and able to focus. This, too, is kind of like a "wake up" call or an instant cup of coffee. It's a mental alertness reset!

Combining cross-crawls with pressing your tongue on the roof of your mouth could be the nice mental spark you need to be more productive, more creative, and more alert. This is a good thing. The more alert the brain is, the faster the body's reflexes can react.

Any Which Way You Can

Cross-crawls can be performed in almost any position that you can put your body into. They can be performed in a chair, on the floor while lying on your back, while standing, walking, or even while skipping.

Traditionally, cross-crawls are done standing by touching the opposite elbow to the opposite knee. This requires both a bit of balance and mobility. However, it is not the only way.

If you cannot touch your opposite elbow to your opposite knee, you simply touch your opposite hand or forearm to your opposite knee or thigh. If you do not have the balance to perform the cross-crawl while standing, try them lying down on your back and do cross-crawl sit-ups. No matter what your abilities or physical limitations, you should be able to find a way to perform a cross-crawl.

Cross-crawls can also easily be progressed to more challenging versions. For instance, if you have no trouble touching your elbow to your knee while standing, try doing them while you keep your fingertips behind your ears. If keeping your fingertips behind your ears is easy, try doing that with your eyes closed or with your eyes looking in the opposite direction of where you are rotating towards. Try cross-crawling while marching forward, try cross-crawling while marching backwards, try them super-slow, try them while skipping or even while skipping and spinning around in circles. You can even try them while eating green eggs and ham!

All combinations and variations of cross-crawls are good and beneficial. Do what you can. It really doesn't matter how you do them as much as it does that you do them.

They can be done anywhere; at work, the grocery store, the gym, the elevator, the men's room, anywhere. All variations of cross-crawls may be beneficial, but all locations for performing them may not. If you do decide to do them in the restroom, make sure it is a private restroom.

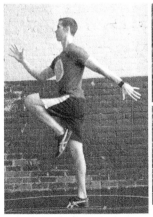
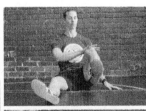
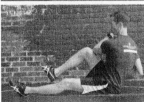
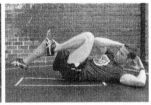

These are just a few cross-crawl variations.

Performing Cross-Crawls

- Cross-crawls can be done in any position.
- Touch your opposite elbow to your opposite knee.
  - If your mobility does not allow for you to touch opposite elbow to knee, you can touch opposite hand or forearm to opposite knee or thigh.
- Explore various ways in which you can touch your opposite limbs together.
- For extra benefit, perform them slow; unless you are skipping.
- Keep your tongue on the roof of your mouth!

Remember, do not dismiss the power of the cross-crawl. This is perhaps the most innocent looking movement but it could have the most powerful effect on you or your loved ones.

Do yourself a favor. Perform cross-crawls every single day.

One Touch at a Time

"In using the Original Strength RESETS, we have found that adding cross-crawls, even while sitting, will help to reinforce the balance and coordination gains we are making in therapy. It is safe, it can be easily made more or less challenging, and it isn't physically taxing to the patient.

In clinic, we have seen some of the most drastic improvements in the patients who have Parkinson's disease. ***Parkinson's is a progressive disorder of the nervous system that affects movement.*** *It often affects walking, balance, coordination and speech. As Parkinson's disease progresses, so do the symptoms. The hope with therapy, is to slow down the progression and maintain the status quo.* ***Improvement is not much of a consideration.*** *However, with the addition of cross-crawls, even while sitting, we have seen patients improve with their standardized balance testing.*

Barbara is a 85 year old female who has a history of back pain and knee pain. Late in 2014 she was diagnosed with Parkinson's. 'I was very troubled by what I heard when I got my diagnosis. Along with my concern of falling, I was worried I would no longer be able to continue coordinating ministry here in my community or enjoy activities with my friends.'

Her initial Tinetti score was 7/28, a 75% disability. Her most recent Tinetti Balance score was 21/28 which is an improvement of 300%! All while having a progressive disease where maintaining physical skill is considered success and advancement is rare. There have been no changes in medication, and very few changes in her therapy program from her previous interactions with physical therapists with the exception of Pressing Reset with cross-crawling both in therapy and at home. Barbara is pleased with both the physical progress as well as the emotional response. 'Not only does it seem to work, it is easy and I can work on it on my own. I have some control again, not many 85 year olds can say that.'"

–Chris Stulginsky, PT
Charlotte, NC

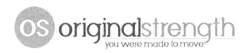

Four Legs Good, Two Legs Better!

If you've ever read George Orwell's *Animal Farm*, you know that four legs are good, but ultimately, two legs are better. As humans, we are indeed made to live and move through the majority of our lives on two feet. In fact, moment by moment we were designed to consistently "Press RESET" through our gait pattern. Walking was intended to be the movement that keeps our brains and bodies tied together. Every step we take should be a neurological and physical reset. But, that is not necessarily the case.

If crawling was meant to be the foundation of our gait pattern—and it was, then walking was meant to be the structure in which we stand. We were designed to walk in strength, with strength, and to strength. It is our gait patterns that hold us together and prepare us to transfer powerful forces throughout our bodies. At least, that was the plan.

> *" moment by moment we were designed to consistently "Press RESET" through our gait pattern*

But, let's be honest, how much walking do you really do? When you do walk, do you feel strength flowing through your body?

> " *Every step we take should be a neurological and physical reset.*

For thousands of years, man has been extremely resilient. He built amazing structures like pyramids and coliseums—with his body. There were no machines. There were no bulldozers, no earth movers, no Ford F-150s, no cars. There were camels, horses, donkeys, oxen, and men. Resilient men with strong backs and legs of steel. Their bodies were made out of iron. They moved, they worked, and they walked. Most everywhere they went, they went on foot, and more than likely, every step they took was a step of restoration.

Yes, they had sicknesses, germs, and diseases, but they also had capability and resiliency. They were strong and they were fit for the tasks at hand. There is a reason Michelangelo could sculpt a muscular statue like David. He saw men that looked like that. It would be hard to pull such a sculpture out of your imagination if your eyes only knew brokenness.

The point is, man was made to walk, and man was made for strength.

Fast forward a couple thousand years. Today, most of us don't walk so much. And when we do, we are not necessarily walking the way we are designed to walk. We are not standing tall with good posture. We are not swinging our arms from our shoulders. Half the time most of us don't even swing our arms. Instead, we slouch, we look down at the ground, we look down at our smart phone, or we keep our hands in our pockets. We are not walking *deliberately* with purpose, the way we were made to walk. Man is not being *man*.

Now think about a lion. They are beautiful, strong, and graceful because they act like lions. They do what they were created to do. What we mean by *walking with purpose* is we should walk like the pinnacle of creations we are: man and woman. We should literally walk around as if we owned the world; with tall postures, holding our heads up on high, swinging our arms from the shoulders. When we walk, it should look like power.

Today, because of our lifestyles, walking is not the reset it was intended to be. As a consequence, we are not as well connected and tied together. This is what makes crawling so powerful. It is more intentional, and foundational.

As you start pressing RESET, and exploring the ideas we've shared thus far, start walking intentionally. When you walk, walk deliberately. Instead of faking it, do it with purpose. Swing your arms from your shoulders. Allow your shoulders and hips to work together like they do when you crawl. Stand tall. Keep a long spine like you do when you are rocking. Keep the crown of your head pointing to the sky. Don't worry, this will become virtually automatic the more you engage in the rest of the RESETS.

Seriously, make time in your day to start taking purposeful walks. Not only can this be a resetting, cross-lateral exercise, it can be a mentally freeing and rejuvenating one as well. Walking can set things right. Walking is intended to be *the* reset.

"But we have risen and stand upright."—Psalm 20:8

Arm Yourself

Before we *walk* on any further, you should know that you do have a right to bear arms. But you also have a mandate to use them; the ones attached to your torso. Imagine with me: If crawling is the foundation of your gait pattern (walking), and if crawling uses four limbs, then walking should also use four limbs as well. So even though we were made to walk on two feet, we were still made to use all four of our limbs to walk.

Maybe the pigs in Orwell's *Animal Farm* were really right from the beginning: "Four legs good, two legs bad." We need to use all four of our limbs when we walk and run. It is imperative for our overall health and ability to retain our *original strength* as we age.

" *If crawling is the foundation of your gait pattern (walking), and if crawling uses four limbs, then walking should also use four limbs as well.*

Using your arms when you walk keeps your brain healthy. It takes the right side of your brain to swing your left arm and it takes the left side of your brain to swing your right arm. But understand, swinging the right arm nourishes the left side of your brain and swinging the left arm nourishes the right side of your brain. Again, movement and brain health have a very *chicken or egg* relationship. One creates and sustains the other.

This is a leap of faith, but bear with me. Brain deterioration in adults is correlated with the deterioration of balance.[41] When elderly people start to lose their balance, their gait widens to increase their stability and reduce their chance of falling. Their arms also barely swing, if they swing at all. But why does their brain deteriorate? Why does their balance start to go away? Which one happens first? Is it because they don't swing their arms? Maybe. Swinging the arms, keeps the brain healthy.

Look around you. How many people do you see who swing their arms, from the shoulders, when they walk? You may see an elbow swing, or your may see a sway from the spine, or you may simply see no arm movement at all. In all of these people you see who don't move their arms, their brain is not getting the full nourishment it was designed to have from walking.

60 Minutes, the CBS news show, ran a documentary titled, "Living to 90 and Beyond".[42] It was fascinating. They revealed some interesting commonalities shared by those who live past ninety. They also pondered why some of those who lived over 90 years of age had no signs of brain dementia or Alzheimer's Disease and while others did. It turns out that just because you live past 90 years of age, doesn't guarantee that you won't get Alzheimer's Disease. The point is, they followed the 90 plus year olds around on camera and there was a very interesting characteristic that the non-Alzheimer, 90 year olds shared: they swung their arms when they walked. The others with Alzheimer's did not swing their arms. This is just my observation, not the reporting staff of *60 Minutes*. But still, it makes you wonder.

Here is the truth: If the foundation of your gait is composed of four limbs moving, then your gait is made for four moving limbs. This is why marching is such a powerful reset.

How to Crawl on Two Feet

Marching is a very deliberate gait pattern on two feet. It is also a very powerful reset. When done properly, it coordinates the hips *and* the shoulders together much in the same way that crawling does. Basically, it is crawling on two feet.

Like cross-crawls, marching has all the benefits of crawling. It is a great reset for mental alertness and it improves overall physical performance. One thing that marching does, that crawling does not do, is marching moves the shoulders into extension. (NOTE: Crawling extends the shoulders, but not in anatomical neutral (standing), and therefore does not increase the angle of the joint and therefore is not technically considered "extension.") When we march, the shoulders are deliberately swung from flexion to extension (this should happen in walking, too).

Going into extension with the shoulders is most important. And, it feels amazing. But when you consider that our opposite limbs are actually

> " *Joy is tied to our movements. When we move well, when we move as we should, it brings out the joy inside of us.*

supposed to mirror each other when we walk and run, the idea of shoulder extension becomes a big deal. If our hips mirror our shoulders, can our hips get into the full range of extension they are supposed to have when we walk or run if our shoulders don't move into extension? If our shoulders are not moving through their intended range of motion, how effective or efficient is our stride when we walk?

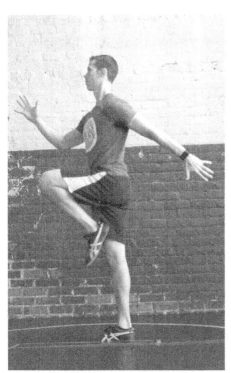

Notice how the opposite limbs mirror each other. The opposite elbow and knee both go into flexion on cross-pattern, while the other elbow and knee both go into extension. The same thing happens in the opposite shoulders and hips. They mirror each other.

Tim is actually marching in place here, but do you see the shoulder extension?

This is one of the reasons marching is so powerful. It RESETS shoulder extension. Which could mean it improves and RESETS hip extension as well. This means marching can help restore walking as the apex reset it should be.

Another benefit to marching is it can also be used to prepare the body for generating and transferring great amounts of force. How many people do you know who decide to go from ten years of being sedentary to desiring to run a 5K at the flip of a switch? This may not be the best idea if the body hasn't been prepared for all the forces running generates.

Marching can be an easy, "gentle" way to prepare the body for the forces running generates. It can help strengthen and reinforce ankles, knees, hips, and tendons! When marching, it is easy to vary the intensity of how much force you put into the ground, as well as the speed in which you do it. If you march fast enough, you will want to run. A feeling of wanting to break into a sprint will come over you. This is a good feeling. Marching taps into a hidden desire in your design—the desire to fly, to sprint, and experience the ultimate expression of your design.

How to March:

Marching can be done in a variety of ways, but we prefer the following method:

- Drive your arms from your shoulders and ensure they are moving from front to back.
- Really focus on driving the arms back to get good extension.
- The opposite arm should drive forward as the opposite knee drives upward.
- Plant and push off of the balls of your feet when marching.
- The rise of the knees should match the height and drive of the arm.
- The arms and legs should move crisply, together.

From marching, it is easy to move into skipping. Skipping is a reset. It combines the movement of marching with a rhythmic hop. Like marching, skipping is a great way to prepare the body to absorb and transfer force. It also teaches the body how to "land" from the small jumps skipping generates.

The cross-lateral, rhythmic, gentle bounding of skipping taps into another hidden quality buried inside of your design: joy. You have probably never witnessed an angry child, or a sad adult skipping. Instead, if you've ever watched someone skip, you have witnessed an unmistakable joy in their facial expression and their body's movements. Joy is tied to our movements. When we move well, when we move as we should, it brings out the joy inside of us. If you don't believe us, go for a skip. We challenge you not to feel good while you do it.

You were made to move and you were made to experience joy. They go hand in hand.

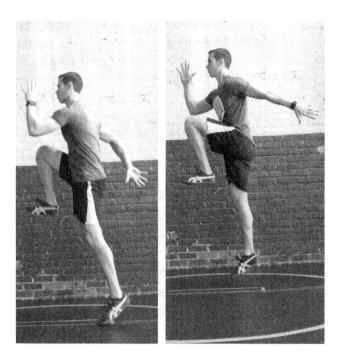

Again, skipping is just like marching with a rhythmic hop in each step.

How to Skip:

Skipping can also be done in a variety of ways, but we still prefer the following method:

- Drive your arms from your shoulders and ensure they are moving from front to back.
- Really focus on driving the arms back to get good extension.
- The opposite arm should drive forward as the opposite knee drives upward, lifting your body off the ground.
- Plant and push off of the balls of your feet when skipping.
- Land and absorb impact on the ground with the balls of the feet as well.
- The rise of the knees should match the height and drive of the arm.
- The arms and legs should move crisply, together.

Express Yourself

The ultimate expression of the human design, the simultaneous displays of speed, power, grace, fluidity, strength and beauty, is the sprint. There is nothing more beautiful than a well connected sprinting body in motion. Just as we were made to walk on two feet, we were also made to run, to *really* run (sprint), on two feet.

Sprinting *should* actually be a reset. After all, it is a progression of crawling and walking. It should help nourish the brain and keep the body well connected. And it can, if the body is well connected before the sprint.

When we move the way we were designed to move, and we are well prepared to sprint, sprinting becomes a reset. It helps build reflexive strength, at a higher level of force. Sprinting prepares our bodies to explode: To create, absorb and transfer high forces at high speeds. In other words, sprinting can help prepare us for life and all the physical impacts and demands it might throw at us.

Depending on your present physical condition, the idea of sprinting may be a bit outlandish to you. But entertain the possibility that somewhere inside of you, there is a sprinter. However, you may not be ready to wake your inner sprinter up just yet. Because of its demands, the powerful nature of sprinting and the forces it generates, you want to make sure your body is prepared to sprint should you ever decide to sprint. You need a solid foundation to handle the beautiful power sprinting generates.

How do you do this? The same way you did as a child. You spend some time pressing RESET and exploring all the other RESETS we've introduced so far. You recreate a solid foundation, the solid foundation that you once had. Once you have tied your body back together, you will be ready to sprint.

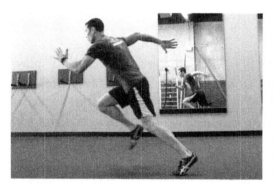

A word of caution:

If you do fancy the idea of sprinting and you want to try it, BE PATIENT. When you are ready, when you have pressed reset enough times and have tied your X together, "play" with sprinting. "Play" means to *explore*. Explore what it is like to sprint.

In the beginning, if you have never sprinted much, start out with *gentle* **skipping**. You can use skipping as a way to ease yourself into the idea of sprinting. As your confidence increases, move into more forceful skipping, where you generate more explosive power. Then later, when you are ready, you can engage in sprinting at **half speed** and work your way up to three-quarter speed. When half speed and three-quarter speed starts to feel really good, you may be ready for full speed! But again, be patient and work your way up to this over time. It may take days, weeks, or months before you are ready. That's okay. Enjoy the process.

Restoring Your Feet

While we are on the topic of being on two feet, this is a good time to talk about the importance of healthy feet. Believe it or not, *you were born without shoes*. Yes, it is true. When you came into the world, your feet were bare. They were perfectly made to grasp the ground and develop into a solid platform on which you would stand. Feet, much like the hands, are full of nerve endings that send proprioceptive information to your brain. The nerves in your feet help paint a picture in your brain of where your body is and what it is doing. They help build a clear, complete movement map in your brain.

If your brain is getting good information from all the sensory nerves in your feet, from the skin, joints and muscles, your movement map will be clear. If your brain is not getting good information from your feet, your movement map will be "fuzzy", or less clear. Did you know shoes can distort the information your brain receives from your feet?

Your feet are two highly sensory-rich platforms that reflexively engage your body. They are designed to support your weight, produce and absorb force, and feed your brain with the information needed to initiate the appropriately timed, reflexive responses you need to stand, walk, run and jump. In his book, *Power to The People*, Pavel Tsatsouline points out, "…another power boosting reflex is called the positive support reaction. This reflex causes the leg musculature to contract in response to the pressure on the sole of the foot."[43] Pavel goes on to mention the *extensor reflex* which causes the leg muscles to fire in a precise pattern depending on how the foot hits the ground.[44] This means there is a rhythm, a sequence of reflexive firing, that happens in the body's musculature dependent on how the foot touches the ground.

Wearing types of shoes that restrict the motion of the feet, and buffer their contact with the ground due to the thick, cushiony soles of the shoes, would be like wearing an oven mitt on your hands. It robs you of your full dexterity and diminishes your sense of feel. It dulls your reflexes and your strength. Your brain is not able to get a clear picture of what your body is doing and therefore it may not respond with optimal reflexive action when needed.

Another problem with wearing shoes all the time is that some shoes are made to mimic the job of the foot, removing the need of the foot to fulfill its design. For example, If a shoe has a supporting arch, why does the brain need to support the muscles created to give the foot its natural arch? The body operates on "use it or lose it". If you don't need to use it, you won't. So you lose it.

Please understand, we are not against wearing shoes. We are very grateful to have shoes to wear when the conditions call for protecting our feet. That, and being barefoot in a restaurant seems to be frowned upon. But, if the goal is to become as resilient as possible, it may be a good idea to spend some time barefooted, especially when you train, or simply when you can.

Having healthy feet is synonymous with having a healthy body. If you want to truly optimize and restore your *original strength*, you need to restore your feet as well. There are 26 bones, 33 joints, and more than 100 muscles, tendons, and ligaments in just one of your feet. There are also sensory nerves throughout all of these joints, muscles and tendons. These joints were made to move, and these muscles and tendons were made to support you and all of your life activities. The feet are your connection with the ground. They are designed to be extremely resilient and strong, just like the rest of you.

CAUTION:

If you have spent years in shoes (what some people refer to as foot coffins), ease into going barefoot. Don't try to run a 5K barefoot your first time without shoes. Spend some time at home simply walking around barefoot. Get used to walking on different surfaces. Feel the different surfaces and the information your feet provide.

A great way to ease into being barefoot is to press reset without wearing shoes. Rocking and crawling are phenomenal ways to introduce all those wonderful joints in your feet to movement. If you are strong enough to crawl on your hands and feet, leopard or spider-man crawling are another wonderful way to strengthen your feet as they do not place the full load of your bodyweight on your feet. Hmm... It is kind of like learning how to crawl before you walk.

Go back to the beginning and you will be able to get to the ending you desire. Spend time restoring your feet. It is well worth it.

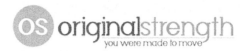

The Guide to Pressing Reset

We just looked at quite a few RESETS. Some of the movements we showed were regressions and/or progressions to the Big Five RESETS; they were easier or harder versions of the five main RESETS. In truth, there are many more RESETS/movements (regressions and progressions) that we have not listed in this book. Do not let this overwhelm you. Essentially, there are still only five RESETS to focus on. These five RESETS are our foundational patterns, the movements our lives are built upon. To review, they are:

- Diaphragmatic breathing
- Head Control, specifically head nods
- Rolling
- Rocking
- Crawling/Cross-crawling/Gait patterns

For now, simply play with and explore the easier versions we have listed above. When you think you have an understanding of those, and you want to explore the rest, feel free to do so. Keep in mind, there is no algorithm or magic combination. Engaging in the Big Five, even if it seems too easy and too simple, can restore your *original strength*. You can become as resilient as you have ever wanted to be just by spending a few minutes exploring these movements every day.

The Neurology of Numerics

Neurology is established through repetition, or lack of it. The nervous system follows the "use it or lose it" principle, but it also follows the "use it and keep it"—*engrave it*—principle. Everything about your nervous system, how your brain and your body are "wired together," is the result of simple addition and subtraction.

If you make a movement, you create a neural pathway for that movement.[45] If you keep making that movement, you engrave that neural pathway in your brain. This is how habits are created. Through repetition, your body will also eventually adapt to that movement through the SAID principle (Specific Adaptation to Imposed Demand)—it states that the body will adapt to the stresses that are placed on it.[46]

Conversely, when you don't make a movement, perhaps a movement you used to make, your body eventually starts pruning those neural connections associated with that specific movement. This is called neural pruning.[47] When you are a teenager, neural pruning gets rid of all the unused neural connections in your brain; it's kind of like "spring cleaning" for the brain.

Adults also experience neural pruning from lack of use. Not moving, weakens the neural connections in the brain. They become "dull" and less efficient, if they are not totally removed. Hence the "use it or lose it" realization. Essentially, not moving and stimulating the brain causes "neural starvation" and it deteriorates the health of the brain.

Not moving starves the body as well. Not only does it weaken the neural connections between your brain and your body, it weakens the tissues in your body because you are no longer stimulating and using your muscles, tendons, ligaments, and fascia as they were designed. The body adapts; the neural connections in your brain, the foundations of your movement vocabulary, get weaker and less efficient while your body adapts through atrophy, weakness, immobility, and poor posture. We are masters of efficiency. The body and the brain are very good at adapting to the things we do, or don't do, so we can remain efficient.

In our modern world, we must be deliberate in making movement a priority. We should prioritize the movements we make and engage in the movements that would give us the biggest "neural bang for our buck", A.K.A. the RESETS; specifically The Big Five.

Engaging in The Big Five RESETS will not only establish and improve the neural connections in our brain, it will also establish our foundation of movement and strength. The more we engage in The Big Five, the deeper, more rooted, our foundation becomes. Eventually, we can have a solid foundation strong enough to support any structure, or lifestyle, we want to build on it. This is the same process through which we built our *original strength* as a child.

> " *the brain is plastic, it is always changing*

This is why pressing RESET every day is so important. We can take advantage of the efficiencies in which our brain and body operate. We can change and grow our brain and improve our body. We can do this because the brain is plastic, it is always changing. Again, this is called neuroplasticity, and it is amazing! Every thought, every move you make, alters the structure of your brain in some way by creating a new neural connection.[48]

The more you repeat a new thought or new movement, the more you cement that new neural connection. So, the more you press RESET, the more you engrave your foundational patterns and reestablish your *original strength*. As you engrave these connections, it becomes impossible to lose them. Well, you could weaken them by not moving, but why would you do that? You were born to move.

Reestablishing your *original strength* is simply a matter of consistency. It is a matter of addition. This is the addition determined by what you want out of your life. Consistent addition is a matter of choice. Whatever you do, or do not do, is born of choice. Whatever you choose, is a positive addition or a "negative" addition. In other words, your choices add up in one direction or another; the direction you want to go, or the direction you don't want to go.

If it is important for you to reestablish your *original strength*, you should choose to press RESET every single day. By doing so, you create the math and leverage you need to restore your foundation and become as strong as you dream to be.

World famous author and coach, Dan John, is often found quoting his mentor, Dan Gable, Olympic Gold Medalist and USA Wrestling Hall of Fame Member, with this phrase:

"If it is important, do it every day."

This is important. Press RESET every single day of your life. It is after all, what you were designed to do...

The Ten Minute Daily Reset:

1. Cross-Crawl x 20 repetitions.
2. Breathe with your diaphragm x 2 minutes.
   - Keep your tongue on the roof of your mouth.
3. Neck Nods x 20 repetitions.
   - On the 5th and 15th repetition, keep your chin tucked and breathe diaphragmatically 5 times.
   - On the 10th and 20th repetition, keep your chin up, and breathe diaphragmatically 5 times.
4. Segmental roll x 3 repetitions per limb.
   - Perform 3 complete rolls from each limb.
   - Remember to use your head when performing the upper body rolls!
5. Rocking x 20 repetitions.
   - Perform 10 rocks in plantar-flexion (shoe laces down!).
   - Perform 10 rocks in dorsiflexion (on the balls of your feet).
6. Baby Crawl x 2 minutes.
   - Keep your tongue on the roof of your mouth.
   - Keep your head up!

The above routine will only take 10 minutes out of your day. It is too simple not to do. It will make a difference and it will restore your *original strength*; in mind and body. You can do this, and you should, every single day.

Warming Up

The above ten minute daily reset can also be used as a warm-up before you engage in rigorous physical activity. These RESETS can make you "reflexively sharp" and enable you to express more of your strength and movement potential while reducing your chance for injury.

Speaking of warming up, have you ever seen a child stop and stretch or do jumping jacks before they run out on a playground? When is the last time you saw a group of kids gather around in a circle and perform calisthenics before they play a game of hide-n-seek? You have never seen that in your life! Kids don't need to warm-up because kids have their *original strength*, or they have a great deal of it.

If you press reset enough, and you restore your foundation of *original strength*, there may come a day when you do not have to "warm up". You can regain the resiliency and readiness to play you had when you were a kid. It is all about reseting and restoring through repetition and the neurology of numerics. You perform enough RESETS and you will eventually create a tipping point to where your body is always ready for action. If your body is always ready for action, you do not need to prepare for action!

Cooling Down

If you do engage in rigorous physical activity, the 10 minute daily reset would also make a wonderful "cool down".

Why?

Because demanding physical activity, whether it be from heavy weight training, intense manual labor, or feats of physical endurance, can take a huge toll on the nervous system, fatiguing it. Demanding physical activity also requires a period of recovery. Pressing RESET after your body has been "through the ringer" is a great way to refresh your nervous system and minimize your recovery time.

Pressing RESET after physical exertion is also another way to add repetition to your "RESET accumulation" deepening the roots of your *original strength*, getting you to the point where you are, once again, always ready for action because you have become bulletproof.

Restoring Life

"I'm an acupuncturist by day, a kettlebell instructor by night and OS'er at all times. Anyway, this lady came to me in the clinic. Patient was an 80 year-old lady with major balance issues having started five years ago but becoming quite severe over the last 2 to 3 years. During that time she had seen several MDs, one ENT and two neurologists. Tests included but were not limited to CT's, an MRI and neural conduction test. All test results were unremarkable. Patient had suffered from numerous falls which occurred without notice and in any direction. She was also unable to stand unsupported. Based on her history I was able to rule out vertigo and lightheadedness. This seems like a reflexive stability issue. The prescription... Neck nods, rocking, rolls, bird dogs and seated marching. That was two weeks ago. I saw her for follow-up today. After a couple of days of performing these exercises 3 to 4 times per day she has had no further incidence of loss of balance. She is now walking easily, standing without support and has even said goodbye to the upper and lower back pain that she used to have. OS has not only given back this lady her quality of life but has probably also saved her life considering her history of falls. On behalf of Mildred (who said to share her story freely) thank you to OS and to all those who pioneer and advance this incredible system."

–Daniel Hanscom
Canada

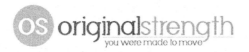

Stretching and Mobility Work

This may or may not surprise you, but we are not big fans of mobility work—or at least not the way it's often promoted or prescribed today. That's because we have both done our fair share of it: Geoff did it almost incessantly for four years—multiple times per day, and Tim did it for an almost similar period of time. We used it with our clients. Geoff's wife, a Doctor of Physical Therapy used mobility work with herself and with her patients, and so did several of our friends, who are also fitness professionals. The unfortunate thing, was nothing good came of it *in the long term*. It just didn't seem to work.

Here's a question for you: *Why do you think a joint becomes immobile?*

The most obvious answer would be "lack of use."

Therefore, we naturally think, *"Let's pry that joint back open so we can use it again and reintegrate it into the body."*

But what if that's the wrong conclusion?

What if we need to dig a little deeper—look a little more closely in another area—perhaps an area that requires some non-linear thinking?

Here's where this gets even more interesting: There have been many times where we have seen, either in private sessions, or in our *Original Strength* workshops, people who have increased ankle mobility *without* mobilizing their ankles (or wrists or feet or hands, if you've been involved in some of the mobility programs we've been involved with). In fact, the common theme has been head/neck movement and head/neck control. Increased head and neck movement (and subsequent control) can increase ankle mobility.

> " *Increased head and neck movement (and subsequent control) can increase ankle mobility.*

What's going on? How does that happen?

Well before we get there, let's go back and take a closer look at this whole mobility-stability thing.

Some have proposed a "mobility-stability continuum"—certain joints require more stability and others require more mobility, where the following definitions apply:

Stability: The ability to resist an undesired movement

Mobility: The ability to produce a desired movement (Hartman)

For example, the knee needs more stability while the thoracic spine needs more mobility. While those are very good definitions, we think they are lacking one thing:

Context

Let's take a closer look.

The "mobility-stability continuum" is a **reductionist approach**, that is to say, one that looks at what's going on with pieces, parts, and not the whole, which by contrast, is commonly referred to as an **empirical approach**.

This gets us back to looking at these concepts from a different view point or perspective—or the empirical approach.

What if excess mobility—or hypermobility—like we often see in the lumbar spine and lower cervical spine is really the same symptom as excess stability (immobility) that we often see in the ankles and thoracic spine?

Based on our work with our clients and patients, we believe mobility and stability are indeed a continuum as some suggest, but they are a *symptomatic continuum* of a greater problem to be addressed.

In other words, the joint-by-joint approach of assessing and addressing mobility and stability is flawed because it is treating symptoms—the symptoms of immobility and hypermobility—instead of treating the root cause of the issue.

The Root Cause *AND* The Solution: Reflexive Stability and Strength

At the time when we first wrote this book, Geoff had a 23 month old son. Part of our *Original Strength* journey has been him watching, observing, ascertaining, and mimicking his son's developmental sequence. This has become the backbone of our regressions we teach in our workshops.

From the day he was born (conceived really) his body was pre-programmed to get him to where he is right now—running around upright on two feet.

What has enabled him to get to upright was what we call the developmental movement sequence, upon which is what *Original Strength* (OS) is based. (Anyone notice the initials OS also stand for "Operating System?" Interesting...)

This developmental movement sequence builds what is called **reflexive stability** or **reflexive strength**. This is what gives us **reflexive control**, the ability to move how we want to when we need to.

127

The traditional rehabilitative term for it is "reflex stabilization."

As the word reflexive indicates, this is strength that is automatic and beyond the control of your conscious mind. It is hardwired into your central nervous system and literally every cell in your body. It's the strength that allows you to move without having to think about moving. When you do have to think about moving, that's a telltale sign that your reflexive strength is missing, and therefore, so is your reflexive control.

In the simplest explanation, your reflexive stability/reflexive strength is your body's ability to automatically anticipate movement—contracting the right muscles at the right times in the right orders with the right force enabling the right joints to move to accomplish whatever task you are attempting to do. This is ultimately what allows you to have reflexive control and freely express your body's movement potential.

Geoff's son does not think about movement. He just moves. Or not. If he can't move one way, he moves another.

This is a critical point: As an infant and toddler this is part of his growth process—part of his ability to gain his reflexive strength. As adults, this is part of survival and we call these "other movements" **compensations**. And these compensations are what cause our soft tissue issues, like trigger points and our non-contact joint injuries.

So what does all this have to do with mobility and stability?

As we said, we don't do "mobility work." Nor do we do "stability" work. Immobility (too much stability) and hypermobility (not enough stability) are both symptoms of the same root problem:

Loss of reflexive stability / reflexive strength.

The reason our bodies lose mobility or create excess mobility is that we've lost some of our reflexive stability and strength. So we are not able to move as effortlessly as we were created; we don't have control of our movements.

Therefore our bodies, in their intuitive wisdom and their survival program, compensate. The body, subconsciously and automatically redirects its energy away from things created to move to things that weren't, or things created to move a lot to things created to only move a little. So we end up with hips that are tight, and lower backs that are loose. Then, if we strength train, we load them with a barbell across the back or a kettlebell in the hands. Maybe we even put wedges under our heels to make up for that lack of "mobility" in our ankles. Thus, the injury cycle begins...

So how do we regain that joint mobility and stability?

Before we answer, let's take a closer look to why we end up with immobile/hyper-stable joints in the first place.

Ever see a toddler walk?

It's hilarious and always puts a smile on Geoff's face. Toddlers walk with their feet apart, and not together. They kind of zig-zag—bounce back and forth off each foot to create forward momentum. Why is that?

Because they haven't fully developed their reflexive stability and strength. They haven't developed it in their "core"—their midsection, the crossroads of locomotion and efficient force transfer.

When they fall, they almost bounce. This is because they are incredibly mobile—not hypermobile—just mobile. Sure, they may take some skin off their knee and cry a little bit, but within moments, with just a mild amount of distraction, they're off running around again, bouncing back and forth, exploring their environment.

By contrast, you ever seen a frail, old person walk?

It's almost the same way. They walk with a wide stance just like a toddler—but without the lateral bounce. It's more of a shuffle.

When an elderly person falls, the results are much more severe than a toddler's fall. These falls often end up with severe trauma—such as broken bones and joint replacements, and in many cases, like a broken hip, with death not too far behind.

What's the difference?

Well an elderly person has lost his or her reflexive stability and strength and the body has literally splinted the joints, by contracting the muscles, in order to prevent movement. Obviously, an older person has greater mass that falls a greater distance. But a baby or toddler has his big melon head to keep from smashing into the ground and that's a lot of work too.

Hold on, that "joint splinting" looks familiar, doesn't it? What's going on here?

Toddlers vs. Experts

Geoff's son doesn't stretch. He doesn't even know what the word means. Nor does he perform self-myofascial release on his baby foam roller. No, he doesn't have one. He also doesn't warm up for any activity or event: Not running, not pushing his truck or his stroller, not when he hangs from the bar in the park. Nope. None of it. Ever. Nor does he use a stick to roll out tight spots, adhesions, or a Thera-cane for trigger points.

We know, we know, he doesn't have your "mileage" does he?

But he has something you don't have—a big head. That melon is the way he strength trains. It's his own portable gym. That's how he gets his reflexive strength and his reflexive stability and why he doesn't have to warm up.

130

Because his head is bigger in relationship to his body, his vestibular system is constantly being stimulated, and therefore so is his reflexive strength—he is gaining and training his *original strength*.

We know you may be scratching your head and wondering what this has to do with stretching, muscle splinting, or mobility and stability.

Here's the punchline:

1. Lack of mobility is due to lack of reflexive stability/reflexive strength.
2. Lack of stability is due lack of reflexive strength.
3. Unnecessary muscle stiffness or tightness is because of a loss of reflexive strength.
4. Movement compensations are due to a loss of reflexive strength.

Therefore, when you understand your problems are really just symptoms, and you address the root cause of those symptoms, your loss of reflexive stability and strength, you will automatically restore your body's natural strength, its *original strength, its natural operating system,* and many if not all of these symptoms will correct themselves.

Over the course of time, when you regain your *original strength,* there is no longer a need for things like self-myofascial release, trigger point therapy, joint mobility training, or stretching. How much time does this take?

It depends on how long you've had those issues. We have seen results in many cases come immediately **and** permanently. Why and how? Because we're not correcting or changing anything here—we are refreshing and restoring your body to the way it was designed to be. Think natural instead of normal. You were not made to be normal.

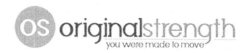

You Must Become Converted Like a Child

Almost all the health related issues adults face could probably be traced to our modern day lifestyle. Specifically, they could probably all be traced to excessive sitting. In fact, according to a recent study in the *Annals of Internal Medicine*, which analyzed 47 different studies, too much sitting leads to an early death due to the onset of chronic diseases like Type 2 Diabetes, cardiovascular disease, and cancer.[49] If you have a creation that is made to move, a creation whose entire design is such that movement keeps it healthy, then confining it to an existence of not moving is probably the fastest way to erode its health and inspire its demise.

The answers to health and strength have always been hiding in plain sight, right in front of our eyes. Children live out these secrets every day. For example, Have you ever noticed how much a child will fight to stay out of a chair? Think about this because it is true. Children have to be taught to sit in chairs. At first, the chairs even have restraining bars to keep the kid from escaping! We use the highchair, or the "safety seat" to keep the child seated and restrained. This violates the child's desire to move and explore his world. Yes, a highchair helps us try to enjoy our meals while it contains and restrains our children, but notice the battle.

Children just *know* that they don't belong in chairs. It goes against their nature! They want to move, to live.

We need to learn from the simple wisdom of a child, if we too want to be able to move and live. Consider the chair, again. What do growing children do with chairs? They play with them. They turn chairs into a climbing gym, a monkey bar set, or a mountain that must be scaled and conquered. Not only do they build their imaginations, but they build their reflexive control and their strength as they learn how to move and climb with the small, four legged play toy we call a chair. Even at the ages of 11 and 12, Tim's children think chairs and couches are parkour obstacles. They know chairs are great for performing gymnastics and stunts over, than they are for sitting.

We also need to learn from and listen to our own bodies. Your body knows it was made to move, and it tells you this every day. For example, how do you feel when you get out of a car after a 3 to 4 hour drive? Do you feel like you could run down a gazelle? Or do you feel like you are stiff and "old". Why do you feel so horrible? Because you haven't been moving!

Here is another way in which our bodies tell us about the importance of moving: Not moving ushers in boredom. Boredom is the death of your imagination. It is our imagination that keeps our brains healthy and ultimately keeps our bodies strong. The strength and health of a child and an adult, are born out of imagination. You know this is true. Imagination gives birth to physical strength; "I wonder if I can climb that tree...", "That shiny, red ball sure does look awesome. I must get across the room to have it..."

When we are idle, the brain grows weary, tired, restless, and ultimately bored. Boredom leads to apathy. From a neurological perspective, this is so dangerous. If we practice not moving, we practice boredom, then we practice apathy. We become very good at these things in such a way, we are no longer good at moving, being creative, having vision, or having passion. Again, this leads to death, or *not living*.

"Where there is no vision, the people perish."—Proverbs 29:18

The Power of Play

Every bit of a child's strength is developed through play and exploration. They do not "exercise." Exercise is "work" adults created to develop strength. Yet, a child becomes ounce for ounce stronger than most adults simply through learning how to move and engaging in play.

> " *you can't take a bench press outside of a gym*

Conversely, adults can "exercise" (work) to become strong and never come close to the strength and resiliency of a child. Yes, an adult can get stronger in the weight room, but you can't take a bench press outside of a gym. Your ability to bench press will never *really* help you out in the world. It certainly won't help you go for a hike on a beautiful mountainside. Yet your ability to crawl, climb, play and explore may give you everything you need to continue to live and enjoy life when you pass 90 years of age. What does this tell you?

Children live out the secret of strength through play, not work. Once a child builds his foundation of reflexive control, through building the strength and coordination to walk and run, he starts adding strength and structure through exploration and play. All the reflexive connections the child has established along the way to walking get reinforced and sharpened as they explore their world through movement and play. The more the child plays and challenges himself, the more strength and resiliency he builds. Again, this is all done through a combination of curiosity, movement and whimsical exploration—it's done through fun!

It is through play that a child learns how to challenge his body, and it is through consistent play that a child becomes successful at overcoming these challenges. This is the essence of strength.

Adults attempt to use exercise in the same way that a child uses play, except adults often leave out the "fun" part. Through sets and reps, adults challenge their bodies and attempt to overcome the challenges in order to birth more strength. This does work, if it can be done consistently. However, for the majority of the population, it cannot. Adults are often met with one failed attempt after another. They fail at exercise because they fail to see through the eyes of a child.

Children often fail at play, but they don't care because they are having fun. A child can't instantly climb on monkey bars just because they are children. They have to build the strength to climbing the monkey bars through attempt after attempt, day after day. Can you see how a child intuitively masters the art of strength progression? Adults cannot seem to do this. An adult wants to instantly be strong after one trip to the gym, or they want to instantly lose 30 pounds after one week of watching what they eat. Because of this mindset, and the amount of "work" (not fun) it takes to succeed, most adults fail at building the health they want to have. Then, after they fail, they settle on the notion, they are just aging and "that's the way life is." Again, this is a lack of vision, it is a lack of fun, it is a lack of knowledge, and it is death.

Please understand, we are not against exercise, nor are we saying that exercise leads to death. For some people, exercise actually is play; they love to exercise. Play can be anything you enjoy doing. It can be a game of basketball, riding a bike, going out

> " *It's hard to grow tired from play but it is easy to grow strong!*

for a run, climbing a tree, or even bench pressing and deadlifting. Play is anything that gets you moving and enjoying what it is you are doing, while at the same time sparking your imagination or curiosity. The more fun it is, the better. It's hard to grow tired from play but it is easy to grow strong!

Want to Play a Game?

Besides building health and strength, there are other benefits to play. Play nourishes the brain, establishing neural connections enabling the whole body to move better. It also helps relieve stress, it improves energy, it releases joy, it improves creativity (builds up your imagination), and it creates strong relationships between people.

Learning how to play brings people together and allows them to develop friendships and community. There is no better relationship builder between people. Play creates friends among acquaintances. Through games, play also teaches cooperation and teamwork, two of the most valuable characteristics a person can have. In fact, playing games can actually develop teamwork in such a way that it just might save your life.

Many moons ago, Tim was a firefighter stationed with eight other firefighters. Every morning they were on shift, they were required to participate in physical training for an hour. No one really enjoyed this. They were getting paid to exercise while at work, but there was no joy in exercise. Some would walk because that was the easiest thing to do in order to look like they were participating. Others would sit around on a bench press or leisurely ride on a stationary bike. There was movement or feigned movement, but there was no real exercise! Also, the gentlemen at their station seemed to all be pretty grumpy or "just there." There was no joy, and there was no camaraderie. Note this: there was no camaraderie among men who would go into burning buildings together. Everyone was there for a job and nothing more.

One day, they decided to go to the local YMCA for their hour of physical training. Somehow, against the rules of the department, a basketball game broke out. Do you know what followed next? Joy. Laughter. Fun. Guys that typically never smiled, nor got along, started having fun together.

Soon, every day they came to work, they would drive their fire trucks to a field to play ultimate Frisbee, or touch football. They started getting along. The atmosphere at the fire station changed. The guys were happy and they all liked each other. Being at work became enjoyable. Going into a burning building with people you know that like you and care about you, is a lot more comforting than going into a fire with people only there because it's their "job." In Tim's fire station, playing games gave birth to friendship and teamwork. Playing games can be a powerful RESET amongst a community. Don't miss this.

As was just mentioned, playing games also creates joy and laughter. Have you ever heard the saying, "A merry heart does good, like a medicine?" This is true. Joy, fun and laughter will keep you young. Joy is a reset in itself. It keeps sickness and depression at bay. Remember, joy is tied to your movements. Being a kid at heart and engaging in play, is a fantastic way to release your joy.

Let's use our imagination for a second. What would happen if, a couple of times a week, you and your neighbors would get together and play hide-n-seek? We know what would happen. You would have fun. You would move your body in all sorts of ways that you would never do being an "adult". You would burn a ton of calories. You would improve your coordination. You would nourish your brain and strengthen your body. You would feel fantastic—*you would feel ALIVE!* You would be overcome with joy. How awesome would that be? Can you imagine how good you would feel if you played a good game of hide-n-seek once or twice a week? Can you imagine the relationships you would build with your neighbors; the friendships you would grow? Will you do it? Will you love your neighbor as yourself? Yes, it is silly. But that doesn't make it wrong. Quit being afraid to act like a child. Live.

Even if you don't enjoy hide-n-seek—and if you don't, we don't believe you—use your imagination and find a way to play. Create your own games. They can be anything, it doesn't really matter what you choose to do. What matters is that you flex your "imagination muscle," have fun, and make play a regular part of your life.

Learning How to Play

Learning how to play may feel weird in the beginning, especially if your "imagination muscle" has atrophied. Remember, play can be anything. The most important thing is that it gets you moving and you enjoy it. You have the freedom to be creative and design your own play sessions. You can use your own creativity and do whatever you like. If you are really de-conditioned, start out gradually. Maybe set aside ten to fifteen minutes to go outside and play a few times a week. As you start feeling better and more conditioned, increase your time and/or your level of activity. The bottom line is do something, move, and have fun. It really is that simple.

If having the freedom to explore the idea of playing on your own seems stressful, it need not be. You cannot do this wrong as long as you do something. Play really can be anything that captures your imagination. Here are some examples:

1. Play dodge-ball with your kids.
2. Go for a walk, or a run, in a park.
3. Go bike riding with some friends. Wear your helmet!
4. Play tennis.
5. Learn how to run sprints.
6. Climb a tree or play on some monkey bars.
7. Learn to swim.
8. Play Frisbee golf.
9. Learn how to walk on a slack-line.
10. Learn how to tumble.
11. Take Parkour lessons.
12. Play Hide-N-Seek!

If you start engaging in play, you may find your imagination and curiosity will start to grow. You may discover you enjoy challenging yourself with your preferred style of play. You may even find yourself doing things you never thought you would do like signing up for a 5k or joining group bicycle rides. Curiosity may beg you to learn new skills and build new levels of physical strength simply because you start thinking things like, "I wonder if I can climb that tree?", "I wonder if I can hike all the way up that mountain?" If you build your "I wonder" muscles up, you will unlock new levels of strength and abilities you once dreamed of as a child. Learning how to play is a great way to restore and retain your *original strength*. It keeps you young and vibrant and it helps you to see the world through a child's eyes.

Your parents were only partially right. When they told you to act your age, they probably didn't know you were always meant to be young at mind and heart. That is how you keep your body young. So, acting your age is only appropriate if you know you are forever a child regardless of your age. Don't let the norms of society steal your youth. Being an "adult" doesn't have to mean you should put away fun, games and joy. It doesn't mean you should resign your body from sports and activities and enlist only in the world of "business" and work. Being an adult also doesn't mean it is okay to sit all day and stare at screens intent on robbing your creativity and imagination.

Do you remember how to play? Get up, go outside and find something fun to do. Whatever you do, don't grow up.

A Simple "Play" Routine

If the previous examples of play are too extreme for you, try this:

Set aside 10 minutes three times a week to "play" with moving in and out of the RESETS as you get up and down from the floor. Learn how to sit in all kinds of positions. Learn to go from crawling to sitting, from sitting to crawling, to standing. Learn how to flow from one to the other.

How seamless can you flow in and out from rolling, to crawling, to kneeling, to standing? How many different ways can you do this? How many different ways can you learn to stand without using your hands?

Just play and explore! Use your imagination. Design strategies and techniques to move and get up from the ground. When you can flow from one position to another, from the ground to standing and back down, with grace, congratulations! You are strong! And, you have just added years of quality life to your body through play and exploration.

I Learned How to Play Again

"I visited the OS site and filled out the form to get the free guide to pressing reset. I was EXTREMELY skeptical at first because of how over-hyped the movements seemed, but I tried it. I pressed reset with the Big 5, and I'm absolutely sure that it looked like a complete train-wreck of an accident. I lifted my feet when I baby crawled, and I was probably hunched over. I couldn't even move in a contra-lateral pattern without having to think about it. Despite all that, after only a few minutes of moving I stood up and instantly felt more free. I wanted to play with Karate again! I started punching and kicking, and enjoying movement again right away. WOW! There was an INSTANT change in my body. It worked like a miracle. I knew from that point that this would be something that I'd do for the rest of my life.

Fast forward about 2 and a half years to the present. I feel AMAZING! Most importantly, I've learned to play again. I feel like I never got to play like I was supposed to when I was a kid, and learning how to play as an adult has been incredibly freeing. I still take things too seriously sometimes, but when I do, I play. I've learned how to find more balance in life. I can move in ways I couldn't before. I can kick and do Karate techniques in ways that I couldn't before, even though I play with Karate very infrequently. I can skip, I can sprint, do front rolls, and all sorts of stuff I had trouble doing well in the past. I can play with kettlebells without hurting my body now, too! Most importantly, I can play with my 5 year old daughter and have a BLAST! We pretend to be Super Hero's almost every day, and my childhood has gone full circle and connected with hers in a healthy way that I never thought possible. I get to pretend I'm Leonardo, and she pretends that she's April and we fight off the Foot Clan together. We play pretty hard every day, and right now it's the primary form of my "training".

—Rick Evans
Arizona

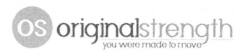

The Message of Strength

You can absolutely build amazing strength through learning how to play with your imagination and your movements. But this idea is a little un-nerving to some. If this is you, relax. You can always build strength through a more "mature", traditional approach. Regardless of how you desire to build strength, it is important you *do* build strength (on top of a solid foundation of reflexive strength, mobility and stability). It is strength that enables you to live the life you were designed for. This is the message: Strength enables you. It gives you the capability of doing whatever it is you want to do. It makes whatever it is you are doing better.

Life has challenges. There are physical tasks we need to be able to perform on a day to day basis to be successful. Every day you are able to take care of yourself and those around you is a day of success. In light of this notion of success, failure is not an option.

Why do we equate having strength with being successful?

Because there will be a day, if it hasn't already come, when you value the strength needed to pick up and hold your own children, when you value the strength needed to climb up and down your own stairs, and when you value the strength needed to put on your own shoes. It is strength that allows us to experience the simple victories of life most all of us take for granted; that is, until strength is what you don't have. When you don't have strength, you realize how vital it really is for success. Without strength, joy, happiness, mental soundness, peace, freedom, and confidence all fade away. They fade away because if strength is the quality that enables you, then weakness is the quality that incapacitates you. Being disabled like this brings depression, anxiety, mental turmoil, worry, fear, and doubt.

You need to be strong because you were made to be strong.

A Simple Non-Traditional Strength Training Routine for Anyone

The following is a simple routine for those of you who want to have a little structure and guidance in the pursuit of building strength, while not adhering to the traditional strength training model. This is a very simple routine you can do almost anywhere. All you need is your own body, a challenging object of mass, and two days a week to train (or two days a week to "play" for those of you who enjoy this).

First, pick two days a week to strength train, like maybe Monday and Thursday or Tuesday and Saturday.

- Warm-up by Pressing RESET
- Crawl on your hands and knees x 10 minutes
  - Hold your head up
  - Keep your tongue on the roof of your mouth
  - Breathe through your nose
  - When your mouth pops open for air, rest!
  - Let's go for 10 minutes of total work. If you have to rest, rest. But stop the clock. When you continue on, start the clock.

- In time, the more capable you become, the less rest you need, until you simply don't need to rest. This is AWESOME!
- Next, grab a challenging object of mass (a rock, a keg, a heavy dumbbell, an object...) and go for a 10 minute walk.
  - Pick up an object and hold it in front of you, if its shape allows.

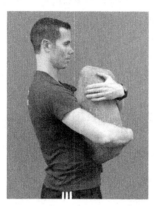

- Walk about 10 yards and put the object down.
- Turn around, pick it up and walk back to where you started.
- Repeat this over and over for 10 minutes.
- Keep your tongue on the roof of your mouth and breathe through your nose.
- If your mouth pops open, rest!
- Let's strive for 10 minutes of work. If you rest, stop the clock.
- Press RESET to cool down.
- Take a quick walk and swing those arms.

Once you can crawl on your hands and knees for 10 minutes of work, while breathing through your nose, it is time to progress! Start crawling backwards on your hands and knees for 10 minutes of work, following the same rules as above.

Once you can complete this, progress to Leopard Crawling for 10 minutes of work, following the same rules.

144

Likewise, when you can carry your object of mass for 10 minutes of work, find a more challenging object to carry. It can be a bigger size, a different shape, or heavier weight. A new challenge is a new challenge...

This is a simple strength training routine sure to enable you to become bulletproof; in mind and body. Do not confuse simple with easy, however. This can be quite the challenge and it is scalable to meet your abilities, whatever they are.

Simple, But So Effective

"After overtraining, my body was plagued by overuse injuries. Other than light kettlebell swings, the only other activity I could participate in comfortably was restorative yoga! I was desperate to return to the gym, but I had to find a way to train that was going to allow my body to heal rather than causing further injury. I immediately thought of Original Strength, so I signed up for their workshop, and then followed that up by asking Tim to program my training sessions for a while!

The results of my training for the past year have been nothing short of phenomenal! I could not be happier! Not only did my previous injuries heal rather quickly while I trained using OS RESETS, crawling, and carries, but I rapidly grew much stronger! My body began working as a solid unit, and strength skills that I'd struggled with for years suddenly became easy. For example, a year ago I was challenged to do Turkish Get Ups for reps using a 12kg kettlebell. Fast forward a year, and I'm able to do Turkish Get Ups with an 18kg KB...and for multiple reps! I used to dread doing single leg deadlifts as I was wobbly using even the 4kg kettlebell. Now I'm doing sets of 5/5 using a 20kg kettlebell!

I could go on and on about all the cool strength skills that have improved significantly after primarily crawling and carrying for the past year. But the most incredible effect of incorporating Original Strength into my training program is just how efficiently and gracefully my body now moves! At the age of 56, I'm still amazed daily how effortlessly I'm able to move about and perform daily activities that at one time were painful! If performing OS RESETS will keep my body youthful, then count me in...I will be rocking, rolling, and crawling well into my 90's!"

–Patricia Olsen
Nashville

Traditional Training Templates
For those of you who are "in the box" thinkers!

The following templates are for those of you who desire a more traditional, more structured strength training approach using weights. Simply use these templates with your current weight training program. It is easy to integrate the principles of *Original Strength* into any training regimen.

<u>3 Days A Week</u>

    Day 1: Reset, Barbell* Strength Work, Conditioning, Reset
    Day 2: Reset, Barbell* Strength Work, Conditioning, Reset
    Day 3: Reset, Barbell* Strength Work, Conditioning, Reset

*Substitute Barbell with Kettlebell, Dumbbell, Bodyweight, or whatever

<u>4 Days A Week</u>

    Day 1: Reset, Barbell Strength Work, Reset
    Day 2: Reset, Conditioning, Reset
    Day 3: Reset, Barbell Strength Work, Reset
    Day 4: Reset, Conditioning, Reset

<u>5 Days A Week</u>

    Day 1: Reset, Barbell Strength Work, Reset
    Day 2: Reset, Conditioning, Reset
    Day 3: Reset, Barbell Strength Work, Reset
    Day 4: Reset, Conditioning, Reset
    Day 5: Reset, Barbell Strength, Reset

6 Days A Week

      Day 1: Reset, Barbell Strength Work, Reset
      Day 2: Reset, Conditioning, Reset
      Day 3: Reset, Barbell Strength Work, Reset
      Day 4: Reset, Conditioning, Reset
      Day 5: Reset, Barbell Strength, Reset
      Day 6: Reset, Conditioning, Reset

Combining Modalities With Original Strength Workouts

<u>3 Days A Week</u>

Workout A: Traditional Strength
Workout B: OS RESETS like Crawling

Alternate on non-consecutive days between Workout A and Workout B.

> Monday: Workout A
> Wednesday: Workout B
> Friday: Workout A
>
> Monday: Workout B
> Wednesday: Workout A
> Friday: Workout A

<u>4 Days A Week</u>

Workout A: Traditional Strength
Workout B: OS RESETS like Crawling

> Monday: Workout A
> Tuesday: Workout B
> Thursday: Workout A
> Friday / Saturday: Workout B

5 Days A Week

Workout A: Traditional Strength
Workout B: OS RESETS like Crawling

> Monday: Workout A
> Tuesday: Workout B
> Wednesday: Workout A
> Thursday: Workout B
> Friday: Workout A

6 Days A Week

Workout A: Traditional Strength
Workout B: OS RESETS like Crawling

> Monday: Workout A
> Tuesday: Workout B
> Wednesday: Workout A
> Thursday: Workout B
> Friday: Workout A
> Saturday: Workout B

Other Ideas

3 Days / 6 Days A Week

Day 1: Barbell Strength
Day 2: Bodyweight Strength
Day 3: *Original Strength*

(Repeat Days 1 through 3 on days 4 through 6.)

Sample:

Monday: Military Press, Front Squat
Wednesday: Chins, Parallel Dips, Pistols
Friday: Leopard Crawls for distance

Day 1: Kettlebell Strength
Day 2: Bodyweight Strength
Day 3: *Original Strength*

Sample:

Monday: Get Up, Swing, Press
Wednesday: Chins, Parallel Dips, Pistols
Friday: Leopard Crawls for time

<u>4 Days A Week</u>

Day 1: Barbell and Kettlebell
Day 2: Bodyweight and *Original Strength*
Day 3: Barbell and Kettlebell
Day 4: Bodyweight and *Original Strength*

<u>Sample:</u>

Monday: Military Press, Front Squat, Swings
Tuesday: Chins, Dips, Crawling
Thursday: Deadlift, Bench Press, Swings
Friday / Saturday: Handstand Push ups, Pistols, Crawling

<u>5 Days A Week</u>

Day 1: Barbell
Day 2: *Original Strength*
Day 3: Bodyweight
Day 4: *Original Strength*
Day 5: Kettlebell

<u>Sample:</u>

Monday: Deadlift, Military Press, Front Squat
Tuesday: Crawling
Wednesday: Chins, Handstand Push Ups, Pistols
Thursday: Crawling
Friday: Get Ups, Swings, Goblet Squats

Reset Your Training

Besides pressing RESET before and after you train, you can also press RESET while you train.

In fact, pressing RESET during your training sessions will make your training sessions more effective because it allows you to recover faster, even between sets.

For example, heavy weight training stresses the body. It taxes the nervous system and tires the muscles. It even weighs on the mind. Once the body is stressed, it can be hard to perform consecutive sets with the same focus, energy, and strength that was applied to the first "heavy" set. As the sets in a training session go on, the quality of the movements can degrade with each stressful, taxing repetition.

Pressing RESET while you train, in between your sets, allows you to restore the body's nervous system back to a relaxed and ready state, thus enabling you to perform well on your next set, from set to set. Instead of losing the quality of your movement and increasing your risk for injury, you improve your movements and reduce your chance for injury. That is the goal, right?

If you strength train, you should be training to get strong in a safe and effective manner. Your goal should be to have strength so you can enjoy your life and/or perform well at your sport. Even if you treat strength training as your sport, you would probably agree that in order for you to be happy, you need to be able to train. So it would only makes sense your strength training routine should be built around quality movements and not merely the quantity of movements.

Pressing RESET between your strength training sets can help you maintain quality movements throughout your entire training session. It *RESETS you.* It even improves your strength, speed, power, and focus while you train, allowing you to maintain quality of movement thus lowering your chances for injury due to training.

Try this yourself. Take a weight that you struggle to press one to two times and press it. Then get on the floor and rock back and forth five to ten times. Now press your weight again. You may find that the weight went up easier, and you were able to press it more than you did the first time. Pressing RESET simply works.

In your own training you may find certain RESETS work very well for you when paired with certain exercises. For example, rocking in between sets of squats may really improve your squat session. Or performing head nods in between sets of overhead presses may totally give you more power to press. This is where the fun of RESET experimentation comes into play. Play—*there's that word again*. Playing with the RESETS inside of your training session is a great way to learn how your body responds to certain RESETS and how they improve your performance. This is how Tim learned how powerful marching is as a reset. It made him stronger in between sets.

From Geoff:

I like to use RESETS that enhance my movements. For example, if I'm squatting or doing some sort of kettlebell ballistic, I'll do a lot of rocking to make sure my hips are good to go. I'll also do a little bit of crawling.

If I'm doing a lot of overhead work, I'll spend a lot more time rolling and doing neck nods, especially if I've been sitting a lot in front of the computer.

However, most of the time, I'll just lie on my back, make sure I'm diaphragmatically breathing, and listen to my body—"free flow." I may spend more time rolling than anything else, depending on my stress levels. At the end of the day there is no "one" sequence I use. I have learned to listen to the feedback my body gives me and choose my

RESETS based on that feedback. The more you do the RESETS, the more you'll be able to do this too. For those of you who need something "set," then this may unnerve you. So just do the RESETS in order. For those of you who like to experiment or "break the rules," (ahem—cough, cough), then this will be right up your alley.

There are no rules though. You can perform the RESET you feel you need. But just to give you some ideas, we'll show you some examples here, done in any order. Some will be traditional exercises followed by the RESET while others will be the RESET followed by the traditional exercise.

Movement RESETS

- Rocking x 5 to 10 reps, followed by 2 Hand Swings x 10 to 20
- Goblet Squats x 3 to 5 reps, followed by Marching x 20 steps
- Back squats x 3 to 5 reps, followed by elevated rolls x 2 rolls each leg
- Neck nods x 10 reps, followed by Clean and Press x 3 to 5 reps
- Strict overhead presses x 3 to 5 reps, followed by marching or cross-crawls x 20 steps
- Heavy Deadlifts x 1 to 3 reps, followed by elevated rocking x 2 rolls each leg
- Sprinting x 60 yards, followed by rocking x 5 to 10 reps
- Pull-ups x 5 to 10 reps, followed by hard rolls x 2 rolls each way
- Leopard Crawling x 5 to 10 reps, followed by a barbell Clean + Jerk

Again, there are no rules here. Experiment with the RESETS and use the ones that tend to relax you and restore you the most. You may be pleasantly surprised to find your movements get better and better as you train, and you end your training sessions feeling refreshed and invigorated. This should be the point!

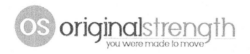

The Original Nutrition Strategy

When it comes to growing strong and healthy, nutrition matters, A LOT. However, If we are being *completely* honest, we don't know *exactly how* it matters. What we mean to say is, nutrition is very important, if not extremely important to how well your body functions. The problem is there is SO much information out there—conflicting information—where experts completely disagree on what to eat, when to eat, and even how to eat. Diving into all we "know" about nutrition can really drive a person crazy. The more you learn about nutrition, the more you can end up chasing your tail. And it can be very frustrating, if not imprisoning.

For example, at the time we are writing this book, "Paleo" nutrition is popular: Low carb, natural whole foods, with an emphasis on meat and natural fats. It's supposed to be the "healthiest" way to live.

But when we were younger, we lived off diets that were exactly the opposite: high carb and high starch, combined with lots of running around and we were super lean.

So is there really a difference in the metabolisms between growing kids and aging adults that make for such different and contradictory advice?

Consider this: When Geoff was 16 and a senior in high school, this is what his daily eating looked like:

6:30am: Drag self out of bed, 100 push ups, shower.

6:45-7:00am: 3-4 ounces of orange juice, 1 multivitamin

10:45am: Mid morning break—3 Musketeers candy bar + can of Cherry Coke

11:50am-1pm: Lunch—Meat and cheese hoagie, covered in mayo, chicken burger (deep fried and covered in mayo), French fries (and mayo), ice cream sandwich.

3:30pm-5:30pm: Wrestling practice

6:30pm: Dinner—usually some sort of pasta and a "salad"

Weight: 158lbs. Bodyfat: Sub 10%.

Note: Lots of sugar, saturated fat, and starchy processed carbohydrates.

Now the naysayers will say, *"Yeah, but you were younger then and you were working out more."*

True.

But at almost 43 he carries around an extra 30-40 pounds more muscle than he did then and he is way stronger than he was then. He still trains 6 days a week, and he is very active. Why can't he eat the same way as he did then? What is it that has changed, besides perhaps damaging (*ahem*, adapting) his metabolism to a low carb diet over a period of close to 10 years? Was it a change in movements? Lack of movement? Injuries? Movement compensations?

The answer is not as easy as it may appear to be.

We know, we've checked.

Again, there is so much information and misinformation in the world when it comes to how a person should eat.

Different peoples, cultures, have different diets because they live in different geographical locations that produce different available foods depending on their climates, soils, and water supplies. To extrapolate one area's eating habits and blanket them on the whole of society is not wise. Think Mediterranean diet, The French Diet, The Caveman Diet, The Frozen Tundra Nomadic Diet, etc.... Perhaps these diets also seem to work for these cultures because their lifestyles are vastly different from ours. Perhaps they actually move and use the food they eat.

> " *with modern agricultural practices and technologies, there are no seasons*

Also consider, in the "real world" there are seasons. People once ate what was available in its season. Now, with modern agricultural practices and technologies, there are no seasons. Your grocery store always has food, in and out of season. Seasons help cycle our foods and give us variety. Seasons also give us nutrition and flavor. Have you ever noticed how great a strawberry taste in its season and how "blah" they taste in the winter? Seasons are seasons for a reason.

Having said all that, we believe a few things about nutrition:

1. The body is made to thrive and not just survive. Yes, the body is great at adapting, but ideally, the body is made to thrive, to live. Low carb diets, no carb diets, and even paleo diets can put the body into "survival mode". While this may be fine for a season, it may not be fine for a lifetime.

2. We were made to move. And, we were made to eat. We should enjoy our food. If it tastes heavenly, that may be a good thing. If it tastes like "bleck" maybe it is okay not to eat it. Life is made to be lived and therefore food is made to be enjoyed. Don't let food consume and imprison you.

3. Even though we said what we just said in #2, you can't expect to live off of Twinkies and Moon Pies if you want to look like Billy Beachbody, or Sally Swimsuit. Be honest with yourself and eat as well as you know how.

4. We were truly made to eat FOOD—good tasting, nutritious food. We were not made to eat preservatives, additives, artificial sweeteners, Red Dye #66, or any other "natural" flavor, or *almost* safe chemical that you can think of. If the food you eat was designed by man to have a long shelf-life, then it will probably shorten your shelf-life. You do not have a food additive chemical deficiency! The closer your food is to the way God made it, the better off you probably are.

5. If there is a "good" food or a "bad" food, more often than not, you chose the label.

We know this section probably does not help you much. At best, this section is really just "food for thought." Nutrition is extremely important in regaining and keeping our *original strength*. But again, to be completely honest, we don't know what the "magic" formula is. We know we need carbs, we need protein, and we need fat. We need salt, **we need sugar**, and we need sunlight. We don't need to live in the land of extremes when it comes to our food.

Again, this may be another area where we should approach life as a child and eat good things (things that taste good) when we are hungry, sleep when we are tired, and play when we are awake.

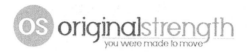

Manage Your Expectations

If you are reading this book, we can only imagine you are not satisfied with the thought of living with movement issues, injuries, "age related" issues, weakness, fatigue, apathy, or just insert any negative quality or issue here. You want more for yourself than just sitting around and watching life go by. You want to actually have "Golden Years" and not tarnished brass years. In other words, you want to LIVE!

Here is a tough question for you: *What are you expecting?*

Are you expecting to be strong, healthy and resilient? Do you believe you will regain your *original strength*? Or, do you imagine yourself sick, weak, overweight, and lifeless? Another way to ask this is: When you "see" yourself in your mind's eye, what do you see?

> " *You will become the way you think; you will get what you expect.*

The answer(s) to these questions is extremely important. You will become the way you think; you will get what you expect. If you believe you can regain the body you were meant to have, you will. If you believe you will end up in

160

a rest home, you probably will. The thoughts you keep in your head get planted in your heart and they shape your beliefs, which in turn determines your outcome.

You might be thinking that we're getting all "spiritual" right now. And, you might be right. However, there is very much a physical truth to what we are saying here. Every single action you make, every single thought you have, actually changes the structure of your brain in order for your brain to become more efficient.[50] The brain strives for efficiency. When you have a thought, good or bad, a neural connection is made. This connection allows that thought to become more efficient. The more you think the same thought, the more you literally cement that thought into your brain.[51] Yes, it is true: Eventually it takes *less thought* to have that same thought! Remember, the brain operates on the "use it and keep it" principle. The more you entertain a thought, the more you cement the neural connection that was made by that thought, and the easier it is to have that thought. Your thoughts can become common to your brain. In other words, you can create *habitual* thoughts, good or bad. These habitual thoughts will eventually manifest themselves in your body, in your life.

This is *one* reason why it is imperative to control your thoughts and your imagination. When you see yourself in the future, you need to see yourself strong. You need to see yourself conquering mountains, climbing trees, sprinting down rabbits! You need to believe, to *know*, you are capable and able to overcome obstacles. You need to see yourself ALIVE! If you are injured now, you need to know that soon, you will not be. Soon, you will be resilient. If you can't walk up a flight of stairs without gasping for air, you need to believe you'll be bounding up those same stairs with ease in just a few short weeks.

> " *it is imperative to control your thoughts and your imagination. When you see yourself in the future, you need to see yourself strong.*

Put good, positive thoughts—the images you want to become—inside of your head and keep them there. Think them over and over. Those thoughts will create habitual thoughts and end up shaping your beliefs. You know this to be true. Think of someone who always worries or who is always negative. Are they fun to be around? No, probably not. How do those people act? Are they full of life and energy? No, probably not. Now think about how those people move and look. Do they move with strength and grace? Is their posture perfect? Or do they slump? Is their head protruded forward? Are their shoulders rounded forward as well? Yes, probably so.

Negative thoughts are "dead" thoughts. Dead things sink to the bottom of the lake, they decompose, they waste away. Positive thoughts are "alive", they have life in them. Things that are alive, rise to the top. They thrive.

Our thoughts present themselves in our bodies and our lives. We reflect how we think. If you want to be strong, if you want to have vitality, think strong! Think vitality, think LIFE! Remember, your thoughts actually change the physical shape of your brain. Thoughts become real, physical things! If you are going to change the shape of your brain, change it for the better. Expect health. Expect strength. Expect life!

And yes, this is also spiritual. Proverbs 23:7 says, *"For as he thinks in his heart, so is he."*

Simple wisdom makes for simple reality.

We know this may not be what you were expecting to find near the back of this book, but this could be the most important chapter of the whole book! If you want to regain your *original strength*, you need to think and believe you will. It is that simple.

It's Amazing

"I used to have neck pain, spasms, tightness, limited range of motion on the left side of my neck and even headaches. I was going to acupuncture for it. Since doing daily OS RESETS since the workshop on January 11 I have had zero neck pain, stiffness or headaches. I have a new range of motion that I have never had before and I can now touch my chin to my chest. It's like I have a whole new neck haha! It's pretty amazing!"

–Artemis Scantalides
Massachusetts

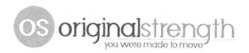

The End?

When we decided to write this book and present this information, our only motives were to learn how to become as resilient as possible and to help others do the same. This is important to us because *we believe a healthy, strong body leads to a healthy, happy life.*

There is a lot of great training and movement information out there in the world. There are also many different schools of thought for the best ways to move, as well as various training systems out there. All of them have lots of great information to offer. None of them are complete though. Not all of the training systems, or schools of thought, get along with each other. It is not our attempt to say that anyone's information is "wrong" or that our information is "right" or better than anyone else's training system. If anything, our goal is only to improve all training systems and movement modalities; to be *ambassadors*, if you will, to the other systems out there.

We honestly believe, and with good reason, that *Original Strength* is the foundation for life, health and longevity. It is the original default operating system, the foundation for anything you want to do or become. We believe it can enhance anyone's training modality. From Z-Health, to Functional Movement Systems, to kettlebell training, to Cross-Fit, to P90X, to Zumba or Jazzercise—it doesn't matter how you want to train, or what system you want to use, we think, and more importantly, we've seen our information presented here will make all other training systems better.

From Geoff:

I have always wanted to be strong. I remember hanging from the clothesline at three years old trying to do pull ups. I'm not the strongest guy in the world by any means, but I'm not the weakest. And at 40 years old, in many ways I am stronger than I ever have been. I can do One Arm One Leg Push Ups, Pistols with weight in the rack, and I'm closing in on the One Arm Chin at a bodyweight of over 200lbs. More importantly, I can, for the first time in my life, jump underneath the bar in a full snatch or full clean, and not get hurt, nor worry about getting hurt. None of those things could I do three years ago, nor at any other time in my life.

After spending the last three years experimenting with the RESETS found in *Original Strength*—pulling them out of my training and putting them back in and comparing results, I can say definitively that this body of work underpins all strength efforts. It is the foundation for all strength. My clients' lives have borne this out. And our workshop participants are proving it both at the workshop and in follow up conversations.

Most importantly, I can keep up with my children—my son, who is now four, and my daughter, who is one-and-a-half. I get down on the ground, roll around, run, jump, crawl, and have a good ol' time with him. That's something that as little as five years ago wasn't even possible, not because we didn't have a child, but because I had a body that was broken—despite having spent tens of thousands of dollars on education to help me become "better than before."

Probably the best part about the *Original Strength System* is that anyone—*anyone*—regardless of age, background, or health history can do this stuff and greatly benefit from it with zero coaching except what they read in this book. In fact, you can do most of the RESETS in here "wrong" and still derive great benefit.

At the end of the day, this stuff is not only easy, it's fun. And isn't that part of life? Fun? Life is too short not to have fun. Especially with the ones you love.

So, if pain and fear of injury and movement have been holding you back, I know how you feel. I've been there. I was "there" for a long time. Now I'm where I was supposed to be all along. It's like a form of restoration. You belong here too. The journey is actually surprisingly easy and enjoyable. I invite you come along. It's fun living where we are supposed to—in a world full of almost effortless movement. Hope to see you here.

From Tim:

Aside from that, I have always wanted to be capable of physically doing anything. Basically, I have always wanted to be Superman. Yes, I am 40 years old and I have never grown out of that fantasy. I used to think something was wrong with me until I read John Eldridge's book, *Wild at Heart*. I now think there is something wrong with everyone else who does not want to be Superman. Anyway, all of us, if we are being honest, have deep down inside, wanted to be resilient, invincible, powerful, and strong.

Why? Because that is what we were created to be. We were all meant to be strong enough to save the day and smart enough to enjoy it.

Put the information in this book to the test. Give yourself a few months and engage in the RESETS consistently. Expect good things. Remember, Rome wasn't built in a day. It took time and consistent effort to build one of the most amazing empires the world has ever known. So it is too with the body. ***Regaining your Original Strength and returning to the Original You is a journey.*** Give yourself time and enjoy the journey.

166

I'll end this the way we started it: We are all, every single one of us, awesomely and wonderfully made. Don't believe anything less than that.

God Bless You.

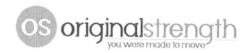

Bibliography

1. United States Luge Association, "What Makes a Successful Luge Athlete?" www.teamusa.org/usa-luge/rules-and-policies, accessed July 1, 2015

2. American Physical Therapy Association, 2013 House of Delegates Minutes, www.apta.org/HOD/, accessed June 28, 2015.

3. Seidler RD. Neural Correlates of Motor Learning, Transfer of Learning, and Learning to Learn. Exercise and sport sciences reviews. 2010;38(1):3-9. doi:10.1097/JES.0b013e3181c5cce7.

4. Sally Goddard Blythe, The Well Balanced Child (Stroud: Hawthorne Press, 2005), p. xiv.

5. Carla Hannaford, Smart Moves (Salt Lake City: Great River Books, 2005), p. 48.

6. Carla Hannaford, Smart Moves (Salt Lake City: Great River Books, 2005), p. 32.

7. Carla Hannaford, Smart Moves (Salt Lake City: Great River Books, 2005), p. 28.

8. Sally Goddard Blythe, The Well Balanced Child (Stroud: Hawthorne Press, 2005), p. 176.

9. Sally Goddard Blythe, The Well Balanced Child (Stroud: Hawthorne Press, 2005), p. 23.

10. Barry Ross, Underground Secrets to Faster Running (BearPowered. com, 2005), p. 62.

11. Carla Hannaford, Smart Moves (Salt Lake City: Great River Books, 2005), p. 111.

12. Sally Goddard Blythe, The Well Balanced Child (Stroud: Hawthorne Press, 2005), p. 35.

13. Carla Hannaford, Smart Moves (Salt Lake City: Great River Books, 2005), p. 39.

14. Idem.

15. Carla Hannaford, Smart Moves (Salt Lake City: Great River Books, 2005), p. 38.

16. Sally Goddard Blythe, The Well Balanced Child (Stroud: Hawthorne Press, 2005), p. 13.

17. Carla Hannaford, Smart Moves (Salt Lake City: Great River Books, 2005), p. 38.

18. Sally Goddard Blythe, Reflexes, Learning and Behavior (Eugene: Fern Ridge Press, 2005), p. 20.

19. Carla Hannaford, Smart Moves (Salt Lake City: Great River Books, 2005), p. 49.

20. Sally Goddard Blythe, Reflexes, Learning and Behavior (Eugene: Fern Ridge Press, 2005), p. 59.

21. Idem.

22. Carla Hannaford, Smart Moves (Salt Lake City: Great River Books, 2005), p. 39.

23. Sally Goddard Blythe, The Well Balanced Child (Stroud: Hawthorne Press, 2005), p. 18.

24. Sally Goddard Blythe, The Well Balanced Child (Stroud: Hawthorne Press, 2005), p. 19.

25. Idem.

26. Carla Hannaford, Smart Moves (Salt Lake City: Great River Books, 2005), p. 111.

27. Carla Hannaford, Smart Moves (Salt Lake City: Great River Books, 2005), p. 134.

28. http://www.theatlantic.com/health/archive/2014/11/what-texting-does-to-the-spine/382890/

29. Deane Juhan, Job's Body: A Handbook for Bodywork (Barrytown, NY: Station Hill Press, 2003), p. 24.

30. Ibid. p. 45.

31. Gray Cook, Movement (Santa Cruz: On Target Publications, 2010), pps. 187-189.

32. www.functionalmovement.com

33. Carla Hannaford, Smart Moves (Salt Lake City: Great River Books, 2005), p. 173.

34. Carla Hannaford, Smart Moves (Salt Lake City: Great River Books, 2005), p. 91.

35. Carla Hannaford, Smart Moves (Salt Lake City: Great River Books, 2005), p. 112.

36. Carla Hannaford, Smart Moves (Salt Lake City: Great River Books, 2005), p. 112.

37. Idem.

38. Sally Goddard Blythe, The Well Balanced Child (Stroud: Hawthorne Press, 2005), p. 185.

39. Idem.

40. Idem.

41. Idem.

42. http://www.cbsnews.com/news/living-to-90-and-beyond/

43. Pavel Tsatsouline, Power to the People (St. Paul: Dragon Door Publications, 1999), p. 78.

44. Pavel Tsatsouline, Power to the People (St. Paul: Dragon Door Publications, 1999), p. 79.

45. Norman Doidge, The Brain that Changes Itself (New York: The Penguin Group, 2007), p. 208.

46. http://en.wikipedia.org/wiki/SAID_principle

47. Sally Goddard Blythe, The Well Balanced Child (Stroud: Hawthorne Press, 2005), p. 23.

48. Norman Doidge, The Brain that Changes Itself (New York: The Penguin Group, 2007), p. 208.

49. "Sedentary Time and Its Association With Risk for Disease Incidence, Mortality, and Hospitalization in Adults: A Systematic Review and Meta-analysis." Aviroop Biswas, BSc; Paul I. Oh, MD, MSc; Guy E. Faulkner, PhD; Ravi R. Bajaj, MD; Michael A. Silver, BSc; Marc S. Mitchell, MSc; and David A. Alter, MD, PhD. Annals of Internal Medicine. January 20, 2015.

50. Norman Doidge, The Brain that Changes Itself (New York: The Penguin Group, 2007), p. xviii.

51. Norman Doidge, The Brain that Changes Itself (New York: The Penguin Group, 2007), p. 209.

Learn More About Original Strength

We have a number of books, a DVD and in-depth workshops to help you more fully understand how the Original Strength System works and how you can restore your original strength. We invite you to visit our website at www.OriginalStrength.Net for more information. While on our site, please also check out our Movement Snax. These are weekly videos of movements you can do anytime throughout your day.

Original Strength: Regaining the Body You Were Meant to Have

Original Strength Performance: Becoming the Superhero You Were Meant to Be

Original Strength Restoration: Returning to the Original You

The Hope of Movement

An Introduction to the Original Strength Resets - DVD

Also look for a workshop near you at www.OriginalStrength.Net/events or find an Original Strength Certified Coach at www.OriginalStrength.Net/find-a-coach.

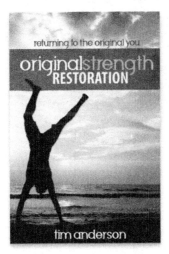

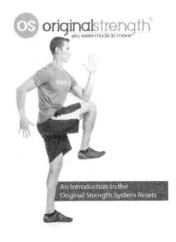

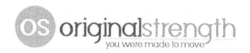

"...I am fearfully and wonderfully made..."
Psalm 139:14

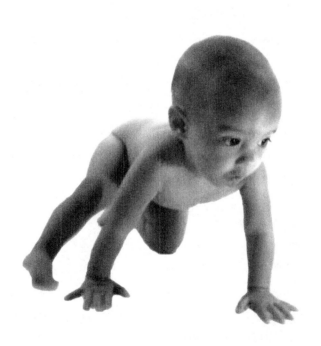

CPSIA information can be obtained at www.ICGtesting.com
Printed in the USA
BVOW06s2238181015

422574BV00004B/6/P